Tim David

Leena Patel

Keith Burdett

Patangi Rangachari

PROBLEM-

BASED

LEARNING IN

MEDICINE

D0318048

The ROYAL
SOCIETY *of*
MEDICINE
PRESS *Limited*

A PRACTICAL GUIDE FOR STUDENTS AND TEACHERS

1 Wimpole Street, London WIM 8AE, UK
207 E. Westminster Road, Lake Forest, IL 60045, USA

http://www.roysocmed.ac.uk

British Library Cataloguing in Publication Data
A catalogue record for this book is available from the British Library
ISBN 1-85315-430-X

Design by Spot On Design, Leighton Buzzard, Bedfordshire
Typeset by Dobbie Typesetting Limited, Tavistock, Devon
Printed in Great Britain by Ebenezer Baylis, The Trinity Press, Worcester

CONTENTS

AUTHORS

T J David PhD MD FRCP FRCPCH DCH
Professor of Child Health and Paediatrics, University of Manchester
Chairman, Curriculum Development Committee, Faculty of Medicine

Leena Patel MD MRCP FRCPCH MHPE
Senior Lecturer in Child Health, University of Manchester
Families and Children Module, Research Project Options and Year 5 Management
Groups, Faculty of Medicine

K Burdett BSc, PhD, CChem, FRSC
Senior Lecturer in Medical Biochemistry, University of Manchester
Director of Studies Years 1–2 Programme & Admissions Tutor, Faculty of Medicine

Patangi Rangachari MB BS, PhD
Professor of Medicine, Intestinal Disease Research Programme, Faculty of Health
Sciences, McMaster University, Hamilton, Ontario, Canada
Director, Honours Biology-Pharmacology Co-op Programme

PREFACE

This book is intended for those who are interested or involved in problem-based learning, either as students or tutors. This includes people who are choosing between a conventional university course or one that uses problem-based learning. The book focuses on problem-based learning as applied to a medical or dental undergraduate course, using illustrations from the Manchester (UK) and McMaster (Canada) courses. Although the examples of problems are medical, the principles and practical advice in the book apply to any problem-based learning course. Details are included of a step-by-step approach to tackling problems in a problem-based learning tutorial. The steps outlined are derived from the Manchester and Maastricht (Netherlands) medical courses and represent one approach to the tutorial process that has been particularly well-studied and developed. The book describes the ideal arrangements for problem-based learning — where there are no financial restrictions; unfortunately the reality for most medical schools is somewhat different. The expectation must therefore be for a problem-based learning course to evolve; this may be in terms of tutorial group size, numbers of highly skilled tutors or access to Medline and other learning resources.

Starting with a brief introduction to how problem-based learning originated, the book then explains what it is and how it works (Chapter 2), and how it fits in with what we know about how adults learn (Chapter 3). Knowing how to design problems and trigger material is vital for those planning problem-based learning courses (Chapter 4). Knowing about how a tutorial group works is important for both students and tutors, as is information about self-assessment, peer-assessment and tutor assessment (Chapters 5 and 6). There is practical advice for students, such as, for example, how to make the transition from a traditional school education to a much more self-directed kind of activity, in which it is easy to get lost without some practical guidance at the outset (Chapter 7). Practical advice is just as important for teachers, who have the job of helping students adapt and cope with the sudden change of no longer being told what to do (Chapter 8). The book concludes with chapters on serious pitfalls (Chapter 9) and a brief discussion of what problem-based learning can be expected to achieve (Chapter 10).

Problem-based learning has been widely introduced into higher education around the world. In its present form it started in medicine and has been adopted by about one-quarter of all medical schools in the US and about one-half of those in Canada, with Europe and the rest of the world rapidly catching up. The method has spread to other courses; in addition to the health sciences (such as nursing, physiotherapy and occupational therapy) it is also now being used in such diverse subjects as law, economics and mathematics.

ACKNOWLEDGEMENTS

We specially wish to thank Dr Tim Dornan for permission to use his annotated version of the 8-step tutorial process, as well as his 'nooropathy lark' case and to Chloë-Maryse Baxter for permission to use Figure 1 in Chapter 6. We are also particularly grateful to the students and colleagues who very kindly read through and commented on the text: Chloë-Maryse Baxter, Torquil Duncan Brown, Dr Tim Dornan, Professor Roger Green and Professor Carl Whitehouse.

1 THE ORIGINS AND HISTORY OF PROBLEM-BASED LEARNING

In 1920, Célestin Freinet, a primary school teacher, returned from World War I to rural south-eastern France. His injuries left him too short of breath to speak to a class for more than a few minutes. This made it impossible to follow the then conventional approach of repeatedly shouting at the pupils and he sought other ways to attract their interest and attention. His challenge was 'to break away from the traditional approach that suited my healthier colleagues so well, and to find a new methodology better adapted to my limited physical strength' [1].

Freinet's weakness proved a blessing for the youngsters at his village school in Bar-sur-Loup, for he created a system in which his pupils were encouraged to take control of their own learning. He encouraged them to be creative, express themselves clearly, communicate effectively, take responsibility for their own learning, learn to be cooperative rather than competitive, evaluate their own progress and adapt to living in the world beyond the classroom; in short, to be prepared for life-long learning. These were some of the key ingredients of problem-based learning, a method of promoting active learning by giving students an opportunity to explore issues, identify learning tasks and evaluate their ongoing progress.

As well as instituting a variant of problem-based learning, almost half a century before the New World reinvented it, he went much further in his classrooms than can be imagined today, many decades later. He promoted child authorship, classroom printing, school-to-school correspondence, project work, semi-autonomous learning based on self-correcting worksheets, as well as open and honest criticism. He was acutely conscious that these changes would have little impact 'unless we change the basic idea of a classroom as a place where teachers are like puppet-masters controlling everything' [1]. To relinquish control demanded innovations that prompted cooperation, creativity and openness. One of Freinet's techniques that he used for open comments and criticism was the wall journal, a large sheet of paper on which pupils could write comments under four headings: criticisms, congratulations, wishes and accomplishments. Erasing was forbidden and all entries had to be signed, so that the pupils learned to take responsibility for

1

their comments. Entries were read out and discussed at a weekly school cooperative meeting attended by all teachers and pupils.

Many of Freinet's ideas would be regarded as revolutionary today, let alone 70 years ago. Fierce hostility led him to resign from the state school system and, in 1935, he opened his own independent school. At the outbreak of World War II, his activism brought him internment for 18 months and, on his release, he joined the resistance. After the war he returned to his school and declined offers to re-enter the state educational system; he died in 1966. His published output was vast. A bibliography of his books and articles covers 50 pages but, although his work was translated into 17 languages, ranging from Vietnamese to Esperanto, only in 1990 were any of his writings translated into English and his work made more accessible to the English-speaking world [1].

RECENT ORIGINS OF PROBLEM-BASED LEARNING

No doubt there have been many others who, in some type of school or higher education, have used something akin to problem-based learning, but the more recent origins of problem-based learning and the use of the term can be traced to North America in the 1960s. A number of medical schools introduced some problem-based, self-directed, student activities [2–4], but the credit for the introduction of the first problem-based learning curriculum belongs to the McMaster Medical School in Hamilton, Ontario, which was started in 1969 after three years of planning [5–7]. One of the later instigators was Howard Barrows; having been responsible for a clinical clerkship in neurology for third-year medical students in Los Angeles, he became concerned that the current assessments were not providing data that was helpful to students. As a result he developed the simulated patient, as a learning aid to provide more data about student competence [8]. This tool revealed that students who had good techniques for history taking and physical examination and who had previously passed excellent courses in neuroanatomy, neurophysiology and clinical neurology, in fact had a lack of basic knowledge when confronted with clinical problems [9]. This difficulty in achieving local change led Barrows to take a sabbatical at McMaster University. Here he contributed to the efforts of a nuclear group who were designing a medical curriculum based solely on small-group, student-centred, self-directed learning. The result of their efforts is a three-year graduate programme, comprising two years of pre-clinical studies using problem-based learning, and one year of conventional clinical clerkships.

The first European problem-based learning curriculum was introduced in the University of Maastricht medical school in 1974. This course lasts six years and comprises four years of a pre-clinical problem-based learning course and two years of conventional clinical clerkships. Problem-based learning has remained a key feature at the University of Maastricht and is used in other degree courses besides medicine — Health Sciences, Law, Business Studies and Economics, for example. McMaster and Maastricht have emerged as major centres for research into problem-based learning, with further important pioneering at Newcastle, New South Wales, Australia. Problem-based learning has been mainly used in the pre-clinical curriculum and a novel theme in the Manchester University medical school is the extension of its use into the clinical clerkship part of the curriculum.

2 WHAT IS PROBLEM-BASED LEARNING? PRINCIPLES AND METHODS OF PROBLEM-BASED LEARNING

The essence of problem-based learning is that a small group of students decide for themselves what they need to study after discussing some trigger material, such as a written problem. After an intervening period of self-study, they meet to share, compare and relate what they have found to the original trigger material and to see if they have covered enough ground. In the process of acquiring knowledge in problem-based learning, one develops a number of other skills and attitudes which are relevant to the practise of medicine (and life). Examples include communication with peers and lay people, working in teams, developing initiative, sharing information, and having regard for others (students, tutors, doctors, patients). Idealism is likely to be fostered rather than extinguished.

TRIGGER MATERIAL

The essential features are that the trigger material is relevant, interesting and provokes discussion. A written problem is the most common format for trigger material. It can be just a few sentences or a longer piece of text — for example, a full and detailed case history. The name 'problem-based learning' implies that the trigger material is always a written problem, but it need not be. Other possible trigger material could be a piece of audio or video tape or a simulated or living patient (discussed in Chapter 4).

Small group

The ideal group size depends on the circumstances. Since an essential resource in problem-based learning is the pre-existing knowledge of the students, the ideal group is one with sufficient numbers to have a reasonable breadth and depth of knowledge, but small enough to allow individuals to engage and contribute. Between eight and 10 is a good size for undergraduate medical students. It is possible with fewer — particularly if the students are well-accustomed to problem-based learning — but a group of over 15 prevents adequate individual involvement. Larger groups are also more difficult to manage and there is a greater risk that the shy or weak student will not participate.

4

Discussion of trigger material

Adequate discussion of the trigger material is essential and there are a number of strategies to ensure this occurs. These will be described in the Methods section, overleaf. The key point is that if students by-pass discussion and proceed directly to deciding their learning objectives, a fundamental aspect of the learning process is violated, short-circuiting learning and preventing subsequent information storage.

Students decide what to study

A key feature of problem-based learning is that the student, not the teacher, decides what to study (discussed in detail in Chapter 3). This has a positive effect on motivation and is important for effective learning.

Sharing, comparing and integrating

Students share information which, in itself, is a skill they need to learn. Different sources often reveal conflicting information and critical appraisal is needed to try to reconcile, when possible, or explain differences. The new information gained from mutual discussion and sharing is then integrated with the trigger material.

Context

A feature of problem-based learning is that problems relate to the context of clinical medicine, rather than to abstract disciplines or subjects. Learning in context makes a link to using the information later when the students become doctors. The importance of the context in learning is explained in Chapter 3.

Is it more than just a tool?

The description above might easily give the false impression that problem-based learning is no more than a method of learning — a tool. In fact, problem-based learning is a whole curriculum concept, encompassing scope and sequence, syllabus, content outline, learning materials, course of study and planned experiences. The use of problem-based learning is often associated with other curricular changes, such as integrating basic and clinical sciences, and it enables the curriculum to focus on issues relevant to the eventual outcome.

METHODS

Students should ideally be in small groups of between eight and 10. For each problem, students will identify a chairperson and a scribe (someone to produce a written output on a flip chart).

Each problem is discussed at two tutorials. In the first tutorial, students cover steps 1 to 5 of the process described below. Independent study is performed in step 6. In the second tutorial, which is held a few days after the first, students cover step 7 of the process.

A tutorial session is likely to last around two hours. The first half of the tutorial will be devoted to the problem initially discussed at the previous session, using the same chairperson and scribe. In the second half, the group appoint a new chairperson and scribe and tackle a new problem. There is no need (other than timetabling convenience) to juxtapose the old and the new problem, and an alternative arrangement is for a session to be split into two completely separate elements on different days.

Students carefully read through the text of the problem. Whether or not this reading should occur in silence or out loud is debatable, and is best decided by individual groups of students. Advantages of silent reading are that it allows individuals to read at their own pace and in their own style, it involves everyone, and it encourages divergence of thought. Advantages of reading out loud are first, if someone is a slow reader they may feel pressured by silent reading and may fail to read the whole problem and second, that the tutor can pick up mispronunciation, for example of a drug name.

After reading the text, students work through a sequence of steps (Table 1) known in the Netherlands as the 'seven jump', a name derived from a Dutch nursery rhyme. Each step is described below and over the following pages in terms of its process, its reason and the expected written output on a flip chart. There are also some worked examples.

Step 1: Clarify unfamiliar terms

Process

Students identify any words whose meaning is unclear — other group members may be able to provide definitions. Students should be made to feel safe, enabling them to be honest about anything they do not understand.

TABLE I STEPS IN THE TUTORIAL PROCESS IN PROBLEM-BASED LEARNING

Steps I to 7:	
1.	Clarify unfamiliar terms
2.	Define the problem(s)
3.	Brainstorm possible hypotheses or explanations
4.	Arrange explanations into a tentative solution
5.	Define learning objectives
6.	Gather information and private study
7.	Share the results of information gathering and private study
Steps 5 to 8 within a clinical medical curriculum:	
5.	Define learning objectives and requisite clinical experience
6.	Gather information and private study including clinical experience
7.	Share the results of information gathering and private study
8.	Discuss clinical experience

Reason
Unfamiliar terms act as an obstacle to understanding. Clarification of even half-understood terms may start the process of learning.

Written output
Words or names on which the group cannot agree a meaning should be listed as learning objectives.

Step 2: Define the problem(s)

Process
This is an open session when students are encouraged to contribute their view of the problem under discussion. The tutor may need to encourage them all to contribute to a fast-moving and wide-ranging analysis.

Reason
It is quite possible for every member of a tutorial group to have a different perspective on a problem. Comparing and pooling these views broadens the intellectual horizons of those involved and defines the task ahead.

Written output
List of issues to be explained.

7

Step 3: Brainstorm possible hypotheses or explanations

Process

A continuation of the open session but students now try to formulate, test and compare the relative merits of their hypotheses as explanations of the problem or case. The tutor may need to keep the discussion at a hypothetical level and discourage going into too much detail too quickly. In this context:

- a hypothesis means a supposition made either as a basis for reasoning, without assumption of its truth, or as a starting point for investigation
- explanation means make known in detail and make intelligible, with a view to mutual understanding.

Reason

This is a crucial step, that prompts the use of previous learning and memory and allows students to test or draw on one another's understanding; links can be formed between the items of incomplete knowledge that exist within the group. If well-handled by the tutor and group, it pitches learning at the deeper level of 'understanding' rather than the superficial level of 'facts'.

Written output

List of hypotheses or explanations.

Step 4: Arrange explanations into a tentative solution

Process

Students will have thought of as many different explanations as possible of what is occurring. The problem is scrutinized in fine detail and compared against the proposed hypotheses or explanations, to see how they will match and if further exploration is needed. This starts the process of defining learning objectives, although it is inadvisable for them to be recorded in writing too soon.

Reason

This stage actively processes and restructures existing knowledge and identifies gaps in understanding. Making written records of learning objectives too soon hinders thinking and short-circuits the intellectual process, resulting in objectives that are too broad and superficial.

Written output

This involves organizing explanations for problems, representing them schematically, trying to link new ideas with each other, with existing knowledge and with different contexts. This process provides a visual output of the relationships between different pieces of information and facilitates storage of information in long-term memory. (Note that in memory, some elements of knowledge are organized schematically in frameworks or networks rather than semantically like a dictionary.) An example of this type of written output is given in the second worked example (page 20).

Step 5: Define learning objectives

Process

The group agrees a core set of learning objectives that all students will study. The tutor encourages them to be focused, not too broad or superficial and achievable within the time available. Some students may have objectives that are not shared by the whole group because of their own personal learning needs or interests.

Reason

The process of consensus uses the expertise of the entire tutorial group (and tutor) to synthesize the foregoing discussion into appropriate and attainable learning objectives. This not only defines the learning objectives but also pulls the group together and concludes the discussion.

Written output

Learning objectives — these are the main output of the initial group work in problem-based learning. The learning objectives should preferably be in the form of issues that address specific questions or hypotheses. For example, 'the use of centile charts to assess the growth of children' is better and more precise than the global topic of 'growth'.

Step 6: Information gathering and private study

Process

This could include finding material in textbooks, carrying out a computerized literature search, using the Internet, looking at pathological specimens, talking to

9

an expert, or anything else that will help provide the information the student is seeking. A well-organized problem-based learning course will include a course or block book providing advice on how to obtain or contact specific learning resources that might otherwise be difficult to find or access.

Reason

Clearly an essential part of the learning process is the gathering and acquisition of new information, which students do on their own.

Written output

Students' individual notes.

Step 7: Share the results of information gathering and private study

Process

This takes place a few days after the first session (Steps 1–5). Students begin by returning to their list of learning objectives. They first identify their individual sources of information, pool their information from private study and help each other understand and identify areas of continuing difficulty for further study (or expert help). After this, they attempt to undertake and produce a complete analysis of the problem.

Reason

This synthesizes the work of the group, consolidates learning and identifies areas of uncertainty, possibly for further study. Learning is inevitably incomplete and open-ended, but this is quite deliberate because students should return to the topics when appropriate 'triggers' occur in the future.

Written output

Students' individual notes.

EXAMPLES OF PROBLEMS USED

Four examples of problems that could be used to introduce problem-based learning to new students or used early in a pre-clinical medical course are described below and in the following pages. All of the examples have the following format:

- intended learning objectives
- the problem that was designed with these in mind
- a mini-analysis.

None of the problems assume any medical knowledge and all would be suitable for first-year medical students just starting their course.

Example 1

Intended learning objectives

The discussion of this problem aims to develop the processes of problem-based learning in a group that is new to problem-based learning. The students are asked to try and assemble the 'facts' into a workable explanation but, at the same time, identify the 'assumptions' that are being made; this is so that if the student went on to study the subject further, they would know what to investigate.

The problem

> **Island people**
>
> 1. In the interior of a remote island explorers have
> 2. recently discovered a hitherto unknown tribe. The people
> 3. appear to be primitive, however, their houses are fairly sophisticated
> 4. structures of broad leaves secured to a base of stones and
> 5. baked mud. Surprisingly all the houses are round and
> 6. are arranged in a near perfect circle.

Mini-analysis

The following assumptions could be made:

line 1	They are free from external influences.
3	They are not as sophisticated or as clever as we are.
5	Condescending; they may be culturally advanced.
5/6	Ease of construction, ease of defence, religious or cosmic significance attached to the circle.

The following 'facts' are present:

Line 1/2 There are no guarantees about external influences because of remoteness or being unknown to us. How did the tribe get there in the first place?

4/6 *Current* structure of housing and layout of community.

Items that might be selected for further study (ie learning objectives):

- seek *evidence* of artefacts from other cultures
- previous building styles
- religious practices
- need for defence on a remote island.

Example 2

Intended learning objectives

The aim of this problem is to introduce school-leavers to problem-based learning.

The problem

A citizen's arrest

You are waiting at the station when an obese, middle-aged man rushes to board a train pulling out on an adjacent platform. He misses it, makes his way to a seat a few metres away from you but collapses before reaching it.

You swiftly go over to him and find that he does not respond to any questions. So you ask a fellow traveller to send for an ambulance. On further assessment you are unable to detect any breathing. With some difficulty and with the help of three other people you turn the man onto his back. A Heavy Goods Vehicle Licence and a half-full packet of small cigars fall out of his pocket.

There is no sign of life. You are not sure what to do next but, fortunately, someone who has done a Saint John's ambulance training course comes along. You notice her feeling the man's neck. She comments that there is no pulse and begins cardiopulmonary resuscitation, continuing with this until the ambulance arrives six minutes later.

The paramedics confirm cardiac arrest, give 100% oxygen and record an electrocardiogram (ECG). CPR continues throughout. The ECG shows ventricular fibrillation. A 200 joule DC shock is delivered through 'paddles' placed on either side of the chest and this results in the return of sinus rhythm in the ECG. A pulse is now palpable. The man is taken to the ambulance and rapidly transferred to hospital. Eventually he makes a good recovery.

Mini-analysis

The intention is that this problem should stimulate investigation into:

- the structure and function of the heart
- factors that predispose to heart disease (which may be chronic degenerative change over years) and the patients' sudden collapse
- the role of emergency services and the basic life support procedures
- a plausible sequence of events explaining how the cardiac arrest occurred.

Example 3

Intended learning objectives

The intended learning goal is to discuss how the human body might be affected by consuming alcohol.

The problem

> **Alcohol on an aeroplane**
>
> A Boeing 737 takes off after a prolonged delay at Rome airport. Among the passengers is a rugby team returning from a successful overseas playing tour. They have been joking with a group of senior citizens, some of whom are very nervous and all of whom have been on a sight-seeing tour. Shortly after the duty-free trolley has completed its journey through the economy class section, an animated discussion among the passengers degenerates into a brawl and the cabin staff eventually ask the Captain to intervene in the interests of safety.

Mini-analysis

This problem could raise the following biomedical topics for discussion and further study:

- What happens to alcohol in the body?
- Is everyone who drinks affected or affected equally?
- Perhaps the delay and cheapness of the drink simply meant people drank too much?
- How much is excessive and would young men and senior citizens be affected differently?

13

- How does your mood (elation, claustrophobia, worry) effect your reaction to alcohol? Are some people always going to react by becoming argumentative?
- Does the same intake of alcohol that makes you a social drinker at sea level have a different effect on your personality at high altitude?
- Stereotyping: did you assume that the rugby team caused the trouble while the 'senior citizens' were models of behaviour? Perhaps the wine drinkers of Club Class caused the arguments in the economy class section of the aircraft.
- Individual versus group rights: should we ban alcohol on aeroplanes if such brawls can threaten safety as well as comfort?

Example 4

Intended learning objectives
The intended learning objective is to discuss public health concerns over food and food poisoning.

The problem

> **A party**
>
> After a party many of the guests fell ill.
>
> The symptoms were quite varied. All those affected had fever though not everyone had diarrhoea. Several people had very bad headaches and a few had stiff necks. Most were confused and restless. One person had an epileptic seizure and two were already unconscious by the time they got to hospital.
>
> When Hermione, the hostess, went shopping to get cheese for the party she made sure she included plenty of Edam, Brie and Emmenthal because she knew how much her friends enjoyed European food. Hermione was always meticulous about food storage and she put all her purchases in the refrigerator immediately, just allowing them a few hours to warm up before the party began. The only two women to become sick were pregnant. Except for one man who was apparently normal, the rest seemed to have been compromised in some way. Two of them were known to be diabetic, one had recently had a heart transplant, another was having therapy for colon cancer and the other two men were taking steroids for unknown reasons.
>
> The people from the Public Health Department isolated Listeria monocytogenes from remnants of the Brie found at the store and the Brie left over from the party at Hermione's. However, there were much higher bacterial counts in Hermione's cheese and the bacteria produced ten times as much toxin.

Mini-analysis

Examples of points that could arise include:

- the guests had a variety of symptoms which looked like adverse reactions to something they had eaten. However, all people are different, particularly this group due to their medical history
- the problem prompts interest in a particular bacterium and the toxin it produces. Does that toxin produce all the adverse reactions and what are the mechanisms of its actions in the body?
- an assumption would be that all those who were ill ate the Brie and the illness was due to its consumption. However if the Brie was kept safely in the fridge, why was the bacterial count so high in the cheese left over from the party?

Study shows that the bacterium produces a toxin called haemolysin and its effects could account for the guests' ill health. Furthermore, unlike most micro-organisms, Listeria grows faster at a low temperature. So doing the common sense thing of putting the Brie in the fridge actually was the wrong thing to do!

Students should be cautious about 'obvious' or 'common sense' judgements; they may turn out to be incorrect.

WORKED EXAMPLES OF CLINICALLY BASED PROBLEMS

Below are two examples of problems that would be suitable for the clinical part of the course. The second problem contains a number of flaws, both in the construction of the problem and in some of the comments made during the tutorial process; these will be discussed in the chapters on problem design and advice for students.

The following two examples consist of:

- a set of learning objectives, as intended by the course planning team
- the problem that was designed with these in mind
- some very brief illustration of items that might arise during the first tutorial (steps 1–5 in the sequence).

Both problems are pitched at the level of a clinical medical student.

Example I

Intended learning objectives
Students should understand:

- the roles of somatic and autonomic neuropathy, peripheral vascular disease and visual impairment in the pathogenesis of diabetic foot ulcers
- the different presentations and natural histories of painful and painless diabetic neuropathy
- the different natural histories and outcomes of neuropathic and ischaemic ulcers
- the tendency for complications to cluster in individuals
- the treatment options for (and side-effects of) diabetic foot disease in general and the specific diseases which cause it
- the role of multidisciplinary care, including professionals allied to medicine and community as well as hospital care
- the psychological impact of diabetic foot disease, the various psychological responses to it and their influence on management.

The problem
This problem is the record of a conversation between hospitalized patients, overheard in a diabetes ward.

Overheard in the diabetes ward

Mr A   Are you on this nooropathy lark as well, then?

Mr B   Call it a lark? I haven't had a decent night's sleep in 12 months. Burning legs, tossing and turning, can't bear the bedclothes touching them. Wife's gone to sleep in the spare bedroom. Don't blame her, mind you. No fun for her.

Mr A   You'd call it a lark if you knew this hospital as well as me. First time I came in, I'd stood on a rusty nail, nine inches long, clean through me foot — didn't even know I'd done it. Had half me foot cut off. Been going to chiropody ever since. Ulcers, antibiotics, X-rays, special shoes. You name it, I've had it — five times. All right for a while, then back again. One time, I didn't even know there was anything wrong till my daughter found me shoe was full of pus. Didn't half play hell with me that chiropodist at the Health Centre. 'You should rest with your feet up'. I ask you. I didn't get where I am by sitting on my backside with my feet up, not like some of these young people.

(Turning to Mr C)

What about you then? Nooropathy? Guinea pig for one of his experiments?

Mr C *'Neuro ischaemic' it says on the letter from the hospital, whatever that means. Went to see Mr Hatchet. Ignorant, if you ask me. 'There's nothing we can do to help you, particularly if you carry on smoking. Your ulcer simply won't heal. You'll end up with an amputation', all snooty like. I'd like to see him giving up smoking after he'd been doing it all his life . . . particularly when you can't get it up, and have the wife going on at you.*

Mr B *(changing the subject hastily). I don't know what you two have got that I haven't. I've never had an ulcer. Mind you, I've had trouble enough of my own. They gave me these tablets — imipramine they were called. Same ones as they gave my father-in-law before he killed himself with them. Felt awful; dry mouth. Felt dizzy when I stood up... took the pain away, though. If you ask me, it was them that caused this heart attack.*

Mr A *That's nothing. For the last five years, I've had to take 10 minutes to get out of bed in the morning or I keel over. Watch out. Here comes your friend Mr Hatchet . . .*

Possible discussion points

Below are listed examples of some discussion points that may arise at each of the first five steps of the sequence:

- Clarify unfamiliar terms:
  'Does anyone know what neuro-ischaemic means?'
  'What is neuropathy?'
- Define the problem(s)
  'I think what we are being asked to do is explain why some diabetic people with neuropathy feel pain while others don't feel pain but suffer from foot ulcers.'
  'I think the problem is all about how doctors explain things to patients.'
- Possible hypotheses or explanations
  'Perhaps it is because they can't feel pain that they get ulcers.'
- Arrange explanations into a tentative solution
  'So different diabetic patients get different types of neuropathy. Some have painless neuropathy and get ulcers, while others have painful neuropathy but don't get ulcers. Perhaps the ones who experience pain have enough nerve function left not to get ulcers. I wonder if giving them drugs to relieve the pain increases their risk of getting ulcers?'

- Define learning objectives
  'We need to find out what actually causes neuropathic pain, and how imipramine relieves it.'

Example 2

Intended learning objectives
Students should understand:

- the pathogenesis of meningococcal septicaemia
- the mechanisms of shock
- toxins and inflammatory mediators.

The problem
The problem is a short account of a child who died. The child's name is fictitious.

Rapidly fatal illness

John Smythe, aged four, was noted to be unwell and feverish one morning. His mother called the general practitioner who arrived at 10.40. He found that the axillary temperature was 38.6 °C and, when he examined John's chest, he noted some purpuric spots on both arms. The general practitioner decided to send John to hospital for observation and transport by ambulance was arranged. John arrived in the accident and emergency department at 11.55. By the time he arrived, his condition had deteriorated and the purpuric rash was noted to have extended to the trunk and legs. Benzylpenicillin I million units was given intravenously at 12.05 but, despite supportive therapy, he rapidly deteriorated and had a cardiorespiratory arrest, from which he could not be revived, at 12.40.

Explain the skin lesions and rapid death in terms of the underlying processes.

Possible discussion points
Below, taken from some actual tutorials using this problem, are listed some examples of the sort of items that could arise at each of the first five steps of the sequence.

- Clarify unfamiliar terms
  'Are purpuric spots the same as petechial spots?'
  'I'm not sure what 'supportive therapy' means.'

- Define the problem(s)

  'What would have been the mechanism of fever?'

  'Does it make any difference where one finds purpuric spots?'

  'What is purpura and why did it occur in this boy?'

  'In pathophysiological terms, why was there such rapid deterioration and death?'

  'What conditions could make a four-year-old boy suddenly become unwell and die so quickly?'

  'Could giving penicillin have contributed to the patient's demise? Could his death have been due to an allergic reaction to penicillin?'

- Possible hypotheses or explanations

  Brief examples of hypotheses or explanations for one or more features of this case that have been offered include:

  'Fever suggests infection.'

  'The purpuric rash suggests a clotting problem.'

  'The illness could have been meningococcal meningitis.'

  'The clotting problem was probably DIC (disseminated intravascular coagulation).'

  'He died because of mismanagement; if the general practitioner had arrived sooner and if John had been sent to hospital more promptly, he would have survived.'

  'The general practitioner should have given him an injection of penicillin before sending him to hospital. This was the critical delay in treatment which caused his death.'

  'It was the penicillin that killed him. He died of an anaphylactic reaction.'

Examples of questions (rather than hypotheses) that might arise during discussion are:

  'Why is it that some patients with meningococcal meningitis die, whereas others survive?'

  'What is the connection between release of cytokines and shock?'

  'Do cytokines mess up the process of clotting?'

  'Was it internal bleeding that caused his death?'

  'What could be the connection between purpura and rapid death?'

- Arrange explanations into a tentative solution

  'He probably had meningococcal meningitis. The bacteria somehow caused an inflammatory response, producing the fever and somehow deranging the clotting, to produce purpura, internal bleeding and shock. The inflammatory response is probably more severe in some cases than in others. It was severe in this case and that is why he died, despite having treatment.'

Students are likely to start off with relatively simple knowledge frameworks, like the ones below:

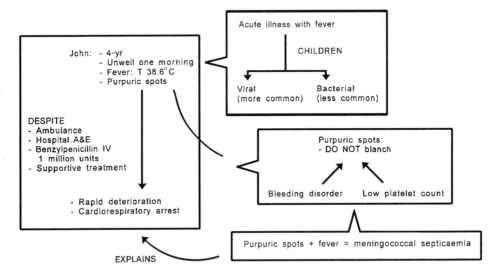

As students progress through the discussion, more information should be added and linked with existing knowledge. Knowledge thus constructed will result in frameworks being modified and made more complex:

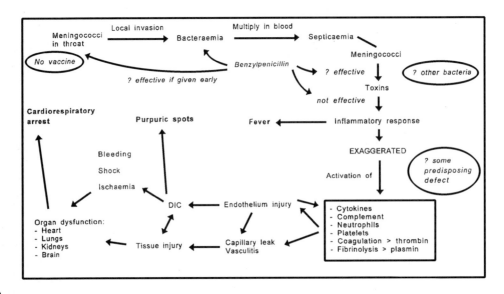

- Define learning objectives

  'What is special about meningococcus? Why does it cause more serious infections than other bacteria?'

  'Could other infections have produced the same picture, or must this have been meningococcal?'

  'What is the best antibiotic treatment for meningococcal meningitis? What other treatment can/should be given?'

  'What is the pathogenesis of shock and what part is played by cytokines?'

  'What is supportive treatment? Is it just intravenous fluids or can it mean other substances, such as steroids or epinephrine?'

  'What should a general practitioner do if he/she suspects a patient has meningococcal meningitis?'

PROBLEM-BASED LEARNING IN THE CLINICAL CURRICULUM

In many medical undergraduate courses, problem-based learning is confined to the pre-clinical years of the course, to be followed by conventional clinical clerkships. However, it can continue to be used in the clinical part of the course, as happens in Manchester. If this was the case then steps five and six of the tutorial process would be amended and an eighth step added.

Step 5

In addition to defining learning objectives, the group should define the requisite clinical experience.

Step 6

Gathering information and private study includes obtaining relevant clinical experience.

Step 7

As before.

Step 8

Discuss clinical experience.

Process

Students should be encouraged to draw on their clinical experience at any stage ('I saw a patient like that last year, but in that case the symptoms were a bit different...'). In addition, some tutorial time should be set aside to report on clinical experience and the acquisition of clinical skills and link in to the theoretical learning.

Reason

While learning is an open-ended process, it will be most effective if students form links between the different components of their studies. This part of the tutorial gives relevance to — and provides an explanation for — clinical experience. Some clinical experience and teaching will be relevant to the problem-based learning case and some will be opportunistic (ie taking the chance to see a patient with meningitis, even though that is not relevant to the problem-based learning case being dealt with at the time). Both relevant and opportunistic experience should be encouraged, because the students must make the best use of clinical episodes as and when they occur. Clinical experience which is not immediately relevant can be drawn upon in future tutorials.

Written output

None.

Role of the clinical tutor

In addition to the usual tutor role (discussed in Chapter 5), when problem-based learning is used in the clinical years of a medical course, there is an additional need to help students identify clinical learning resources. This may be advice as to where to find patients with certain problems, suggestions as to resources that are available in the community, or advice about the suitability and availability of medical and paramedical personnel.

3 HOW ADULTS LEARN AND HOW THIS APPLIES TO PROBLEM-BASED LEARNING

Figure 1 shows two boys in their school playground with their teacher. The teacher decides what the boys do for each lesson, which books they read, corrects any mistakes they make, sets their homework and provides and marks any tests. She also supervises them at lunch and helps them if they have trouble changing their clothes or tying up shoe-laces.

The boys are very happy with this arrangement, but would adults like to be dressed up in a school uniform and treated in this way? Of course not. Adults are not just large children but, unfortunately, the way children are taught is the only style of education many people know, for it has dominated school, and even adult,

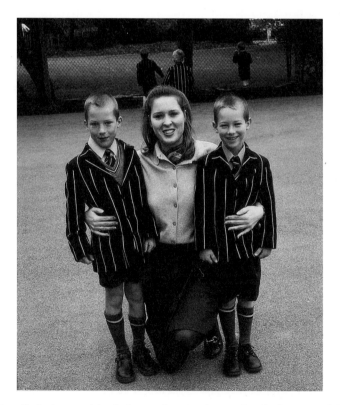

Figure 1   Two little boys with their teacher in their school playground. Reproduced with permission from the *Journal of the Royal Society of Medicine*

education until recently. Below we have summarized the main differences between a stereotyped traditional pedagogy (child-learning) and the model that is predicted by the adult learning theory [10]. Looking at the differences between the two models, it is plain that the conventional, undergraduate, lecture-based curriculum fits best with the educational needs of a small child. It is, therefore, not surprising that there is currently a great deal of interest being shown in problem-based learning as an alternative.

CHILD-CENTRED VERSUS ADULT LEARNING MODEL

Dependent learning

In the traditional learning model, the learner is a dependent person who submissively carries out the teacher's directions. In the adult learning model, the learner is self-directing. Conditioned at school (or by social situations) to assume a role of dependency, adults (eg the recent school leaver or the adult who has never learnt to be self-directed) sometimes demand to be taught. Thus adults need to make a transition from the comfort of being dependent to being self-directed.

Adults need to be seen as being capable of taking responsibility for themselves. When adults feel that others are imposing their wills, there may be resentment and resistance.

Readiness to learn

In the traditional learning model, the person becomes ready to learn what they are told they should learn in order to advance to the next grade level. Readiness to learn is largely a function of age. In contrast, adults become ready to learn when they experience a need to know or do something — readiness develops naturally. Things can be done to induce it, such as exposing learners to more effective role models or to diagnostic experiences in which they can assess gaps between where they are and where they want to be.

Role of the learner's experience

In the traditional learning model, learners are assumed to enter with little experience that is of value as a resource in learning. It is the experience of the teacher, the textbook writer or the audio-visual aids producer that counts. Learning is based on transmission techniques — lectures, assigned reading and audio-visual presentations. By contrast, adults enter with a greater volume and a different quality of experience from youth and are themselves a rich resource for one another. Adults also have a stronger sense of self-identity based on their life experience. So if in an educational situation an adult's experience is ignored, or criticized, it is not just the experience that is being rejected — it is the person. Hence the importance of using adult experience as a learning resource. The negative consequence of adulthood is that, because of their experience, adults often have developed habitual ways of thinking and acting, preconceptions about reality and prejudices or defensiveness about former ways of thinking and doing. Adult learners frequently need help to become more open-minded.

Orientation to learning

In the traditional learning model, learners are subject-orientated. They see learning as a process of being taught carefully prescribed content matter. The curriculum is organized according to subjects. On the other hand, adults enter with a life-centred, task-centred or problem-centred orientation to learning. For adult learners, learning experiences need to be orientated to life rather than to subject matter.

Motivation to learn

In the traditional learning model, learners are motivated primarily by external pressures from parents and teachers, competition for grades and the consequences of failure. Although adults also respond to these external motivators and others — such as a better job and salary increase — the adult model predicts that more potent motivators will be internal: self-esteem, recognition, better quality of life, greater self-confidence.

CONTRASTING MODELS: A NOTE OF CAUTION

Although for centuries we had only the traditional learning model, it is clear that there are now two sets of assumptions about learners. In relation to the comparisons between these two models, some notes of caution are needed.

Stereotypes

The two models are deliberately stereotyped, to make the contrast obvious. However the adult learning model does not imply that the stereotyped, traditional learning model is either appropriate or best practice for children of all ages.

The adult learning model sometimes applies to children

The adult learning model applies to children more than we think. For instance, children are very self-directed outside school (for example when playing), and are capable of being self-directed in school.

Adult learners sometimes need to be dependent

In some situations, such as when learners enter a totally strange territory, they may be wholly dependent on didactic instruction before they can take much initiative.

Models fail to include 'adolescence'

The two models are deliberately polarized into two extremes of 'child' and 'adult'. It is clear that in real life the transition from school child to self-directed adult learner is a gradual process, passing through a sort of educational 'adolescence'. It is misleading to think that school children can become adult learners overnight; it takes time.

HOW DO WE LEARN AND STORE NEW INFORMATION?

It is possible to cram huge amounts of information into the human brain — this is how we authors passed our anatomy, physiology and biochemistry examinations. However, much of this information is rapidly lost; after the examination the cerebral hard disc is wiped clean, ready for the next course and its examination.

As a result of a number of experiments, we know that learning is an active rather than a passive process, and there are a number of prerequisites for the storage of a new item of information. These are listed below and opposite.

New information must be glued on to existing stored information

A new piece of information can only be stored long-term by being glued on to a piece of information already existing in the memory. Loose facts have nowhere to go and are lost.

Old information must be taken out and dusted for glue to be applied

Adhesion between the new and old pieces of information can only occur if the old information has been retrieved from the memory, and cleaned and dusted (ie thought about and maybe modified).

Contextual information is stored with new information

When new information is stored, simultaneous storage of information about the context also takes place. This contextual information could be relevant to a clinical problem (eg how chickenpox spread from one child to other patients on the ward) or irrelevant (eg you saw the patient on the day England won the world cup). When remembering details of a patient in hospital, one is likely to also remember apparently irrelevant information such as the colour of the hair or the location of the bed on the ward. Contextual information is important; it is much harder to recall information when one is in a different context. This explains why when you meet someone from work at the shops you suddenly cannot remember their name. Transfer of knowledge from one situation to another is generally very poor [11]. The more a new situation resembles an old situation, the better the transfer will be [12]. This is one of the reasons that the context provided by problems or cases is important [13]. Relevant contextual knowledge is a prerequisite for understanding information. The greater the understanding, the better the storage of the information. Providing variable but relevant contexts is important for learning. An example of variable but relevant contexts might be discussing a case of meningococcal septicaemia in a tutorial, seeing a case on a ward round, seeing a patient with a petechial or purpuric rash in general practice, and reading about it after doing a search of the library.

RELATIONSHIP WITH PROBLEM-BASED LEARNING

Learning is an active process, and the 7- or 8-steps of the problem-based learning process fit well with what we know about the storage and subsequent retrieval of new information. It also fits well with our knowledge on how adults learn. In

27

problem-based learning, the student decides on his or her own learning objectives as a result of exposure to trigger material (eg a written problem, a video or a patient). The role of the teacher is to design trigger material that will interest and hold the attention of the student, motivate the student to learn, and to provide the appropriate learning resources (eg library materials, computerized literature searching, video materials, skills laboratories, clinical exposure). Other than the design and provision of the trigger material, the whole educational process is in the control of the student.

4 PROBLEM AND TRIGGER MATERIAL DESIGN

FROM FACULTY LEARNING OBJECTIVES TO STUDENT LEARNING OBJECTIVES

Designing problems involves the following sequence — a feedback loop:

- The module design team selects one or more learning objectives.
- The module design team constructs a problem, with the aim that use of this problem by students will lead them to choose learning objectives broadly similar to the ones the design team had in mind.
- If possible, the problem is piloted by a group of students before it is introduced into the module.
- Students use the problem. In the course of doing so, they choose learning objectives.
- The tutor feeds back these learning objectives to the module design team. If the learning objectives of the students were similar to those of the module designer, the problem can be re-used when the module is used by future students. If the students selected learning objectives that differed importantly from those that were intended, then the module design team make changes to the problem or scrap it altogether.

GOOD PROBLEMS ARE ESSENTIAL

Problems stimulate students to learn in their tutorial groups and independently. The quality of the problems influences group functioning, students' individual study time, interest in the subject matter and achievement [14]. The content of a problem indirectly guides students to the intended learning objectives and corresponding learning activities. Some variation in the type of problems presented in a course helps to maintain students' interest and engagement.

PROBLEMS SHOULD FIT THE COURSE DESIGN

Problems need to be tailored to their position in a course and the sequencing of material within the course.

29

PROBLEMS SHOULD BE AT THE RIGHT LEVEL OF ORGANIZATION

Depending on the educational goal, problems may vary in format and may be designed at different levels of human functioning eg cell, tissue, organ, system, person, family or community.

NORMAL OR PATHOLOGICAL?

At each level, the problem may depict normal functioning or abnormal (pathological) functioning, depending on the place in the curriculum and the intended objectives.

NEED FOR COURSE OUTLINE FOR PROBLEM DESIGNERS

A course outline is crucial before problems are designed. The course outline contains the major ideas, components or topics for learning. A concise course outline is needed to identify intended learning objectives. As it is impossible to accommodate 'everything' into any curriculum, one has to establish priorities by using, for example, expert consensus and indices of educational importance such as:

- incidence and prevalence of a condition according to community health statistics
- severity of a condition: emergencies, life threatening conditions, significant adverse effects on life
- accuracy and predictive value of diagnostic tests
- the feasibility of monitoring quality of care
- conditions amenable to intervention, beneficial interventions: preventable conditions, treatable conditions, rehabilitative measures, significant benefit if quality of life is improved
- conditions requiring interdisciplinary input
- conditions emphasizing basic concepts and ideas
- prototypicality.

PROBLEM COMPONENTS

A problem consists of a title and a body of text or audio-visual material. Although guiding questions may be added in order to focus attention, they risk pre-empting the learning agenda and can compromise students' interest for exploring and discovering.

Guiding questions are particularly useful at the beginning of a problem-based learning course, when one is trying to help students make the transition from a traditional school education to being self-directed. For example, in the problem below, which is useful for introducing people to problem-based learning, the guiding question is essential.

Thunderclap problem

It is a hot and humid day. Many ascending dust particles can be observed in the air. By the end of the afternoon, dark clouds are building up and the weather becomes even more sultry. Then, suddenly, lightning in the far distance followed by a thunderclap. Heavy rain. A thunderstorm.

Explain these phenomena.

Sometimes a guiding question is helpful, even if the problem is to be used by students who are familiar with problem-based learning.

A busy day

On the same day in the clinic you meet two patients, both of whom have recently experienced a road traffic accident. They have been injured, but not seriously.

— Miss A's accident was five days earlier. She complains of not being able to eat or sleep. Attacks of shaking and crying are overwhelming her.

— Mr P's accident was the night before. He was very active, talking incessantly but clearly quite concerned about the impact of what had happened.

Explain why they were so different in their reactions.

PROBLEM FORMATS

Problem formats may be classified into at least eight different categories described overleaf [15].

I. The story

The story is a description of a situation or event. Generally, a patient figure as the central character and the story resembles the traditional clinical case. It may be presented as a paper case, by a real or simulated patient, or by a video recording.

The story format encourages students to explain symptoms and findings and, in the clinical years, to diagnose. It can emphasize the elaboration of clinical knowledge. For example, the text of a problem might include 'The patient was cyanosed but not clubbed.' The following discussion might follow:

A. 'I thought that if people were cyanosed they were also clubbed.'
B. 'No, you only get clubbing if the problem is chronic.'
C. 'How long does the condition have to exist for clubbing to develop? Weeks? Months? Years?'

To make the material more lifelike, and because students may well model the format for their own patient record keeping, it is helpful to present all laboratory data (including normal ranges) in a case rather than merely selecting a few abnormal results.

A useful type of story format is the use of edited correspondence (with the real names changed). If the intended learning objectives focus on normal pregnancy and what happens when an expectant mother first visits the hospital, then the trigger material might comprise a general practitioner's letter of referral of a pregnant woman to the hospital. If the intended learning objectives focus on a child psychiatry problem, then the trigger material might consist of a series of letters about a child written by a general practitioner, a hospital paediatrician, and the child psychiatrist. Letters do not always have to be written by doctors. In a psychosexual problem, one might use a letter written to a newspaper 'agony aunt'. In a case that focused on obstetric care before and during delivery, or on the causes of handicap, the trigger material might be a letter from a solicitor claiming negligence against the hospital. 'Overheard conversations' (as in the 'nooropathy lark' case (chapter 2)) are another lifelike and stimulating way to present material.

2. The SOAP case

The SOAP case is a description of a patient case according to a specific format. SOAP refers to:

Subjective (information given to the physician by the patient)
Objective (information gathered by the physician by means of physical examination)

Assessment (the set of working diagnoses)

Plan (management plan in terms of investigations, treatment and follow-up).

3. The Problem Oriented Medical Record

The Problem Oriented Medical Record is also a description of a patient case according to a specific format which starts by identifying and listing all the patient's problems (including medical and social). It is a systematic approach to the complaint(s) presented to the physician and the associated underlying physical, mental or social problems.

The SOAP case and Problem Oriented Medical Record trigger students to reflect, think and deliberate about what enquiries (eg in the history), observations (eg examination findings) or investigations should be made to obtain further information and about diagnoses and management.

4. The segmented progressive disclosure problem

The segmented progressive disclosure problem is a format in which the problem is presented as several segments in different sessions, either as handouts containing information, correspondence letters, video recordings or simulated/real patient encounters. This simulates the step-wise acquisition of data and the successive formulations that typically occur in real life practice. Each new hypothesis is based on new data, each stimulates a new phase of enquiry, and each increment of scientific knowledge then contributes to understanding clinical issues. As the problem is split into segments, it avoids overwhelming the student with too much data at the outset.

5. The problem package

The problem package is a format in which similar problems are grouped together. Similarity may pertain to a main complaint such as chest pain or a pathophysiological state such as cardiac failure (but with different underlying causes or diagnoses), or to a diagnosis such as diabetes mellitus (but with different presentations, complaints or management options).

The following is an example of a problem package format:

33

Children with heart problems

Connie was found to have a heart murmur during the routine six-week baby check-up. There were no abnormalities on examination of the cardiovascular system apart from a grade 2/6 ejection systolic murmur maximal in the second left intercostal space.

Sam was born by normal delivery at term. When he was 30-minutes-old, a routine examination by the SHO revealed a grade 4/6 pansytolic murmur all over the praecordium and back. There was no thrill and there were no other abnormal findings. The parents were very worried as their first baby died of a heart defect when she was only one-week-old.

When Megan was seven-days-old, she was found to be pale and limp after a feed. Her parents thought she was dying and rushed her to hospital. On examination she was found to be pale, clammy, lethargic and floppy. Her respiratory rate was 80/min. Her right brachial pulse was palpable, pulse rate 180/min. The left brachial pulse and the femoral pulses could not be felt. There was no murmur.

Callum is an eight-year-old with Down's syndrome. On examination, he is noted to have blue lips and mucous membranes, finger clubbing, shortness of breath, bulging left anterior hemithorax, pulse rate 90/min, and a grade 2/6 ejection systolic murmur in the second left intercostal space.

The problem package format draws students' attention to the clinical aspects of disease and the pitfalls in medical practice that physicians must be prepared for. Students learn to identify conditions that look alike but that have quite different underlying mechanisms and consequently require different management. Students also learn the different features and outcomes of the same condition.

6. The phenomenon

The phenomenon is a short outline of one or more observations made without offering a description of a real patient, the pertaining backgrounds or medical history. This format triggers students to discuss and explain in terms of basic science knowledge.

The following is an example of a problem using phenomena:

> **Cold hands**
>
> *Johnny Green, seven-years-old, is playing bare-handed in the snow on a beautiful clear winter day. After a while, he notices that his hands have become quite cold and look pale. By the time Johnny arrives home crying, his hands have turned blue. 'My hands are so cold' he tells his mother. Despite Johnny's loud protest, his mother holds his hands under the cold water tap. 'Feeling better?' she asks after a while. 'They are glowing', Johnny replies. 'It feels like a million needles pricking'.*
>
> *Explain these phenomena in terms of underlying processes.*

7. Drawings

Drawings, for example of a neurological pathway, or a flow chart can serve as triggers that help integrate clinical knowledge with biomedical knowledge. Other visual formats can also serve a similar purpose.

8. A strategy task

Problems with this format require an action component, for example 'Design an antenatal information sheet' or 'Write an information sheet for parents of a child who has had a febrile convulsion'. It may require students to conduct a survey or interview, or to indicate how they might act in a particular situation.

SPECIFIC DESIGN FEATURES

Problem designers need insight into students' existing knowledge

Students use their prior/existing knowledge to discuss and explain the phenomena presented in a problem. Thus, the problem should match the level of knowledge students already have and should contain cues to activate memory of existing knowledge. This implies that problem designers need to have insight into students' prior/existing knowledge.

The problem must be relevant

New students come from an examination culture, and are apt to think of relevance as referring to the content of the next examination. From the viewpoint of problem-based learning, anything that aids the processes of understanding and deep learning is relevant. A relevant realistic problem arouses curiosity, is intrinsically motivating for students and will encourage further study activities. Relating new knowledge to existing knowledge and learning in the functional context in which it will subsequently be applied assists students to organize long-term memory for ready retrieval. Thus, the problem should deal with situations that can be expected to occur in the students' future professional practice. For medical curricula, the problems should reflect a real-life situation (an example of an event that has actually happened or could happen) in terms of incidence, seriousness, preventability, clinical situations, practitioner and patient profiles. Students should be able to recognize the relevance of the problem with regard to professional practice. Although realistic, the problem should not include too many distractors. Distractors are items or cues that are not necessary and are not linked to intended learning objectives. Distractors, sometimes put in as deliberate red herrings, can simply build up to become insurmountable hurdles to learning.

The problem should be striking

The problem should attempt to leave at least one vivid image that impresses itself on the students' memories and that will serve as a key to open the door of more specific recollections.

The problem should neither be too easy nor too complex

The problem should help students focus on the intended purpose. At the same time it should not be so obvious that students do not have to think for themselves: it should leave wide enough scope for exploration.

The problem should be feasible

The problem should be open enough to sustain discussion about possible solutions. It should be feasible to discuss the problem within the specified duration of the tutorial.

The effect on the student should be considered

The problem should lead students in the direction of the faculty's educational objectives. It should be a stimulus for studying relevant basic concepts and integrating concepts from different disciplines.

Problem designers need to consider whether or not the learning goals that students formulate after working on a problem will result in appropriate self-study activities. The problem should direct and focus learning towards a limited number of prioritized issues. Long and highly complex cases that embrace a large number of issues and call for a wide breadth of clinical reasoning tend to sacrifice depth. Trying to brainstorm 25 different topics in 60 minutes makes it impossible to look at any topic in any useful detail.

The time available to the student should be considered

When the workload required to adequately address learning issues exceeds the maximum reasonable time available for students to spend on the task, they will adapt by using minimalist (surface) approaches. Examples of the latter are taking 'short-cuts' such as copying notes from other students or directly from books, and skipping important learning activities. A more subtle effect of excessive workload may be that students shift their major intention away from understanding to one of simply avoiding failure in examinations.

The problem should be short

There are several advantages to keeping problems relatively short. The longer the problem, the greater the scope for students to 'go off at a tangent' and miss the key intended learning issues. Long problems make it more difficult to focus on a few selected topics or explore issues in depth. They may also lead to a large number of topics for discussion, leaving less time for brainstorming or hypothesis generation, and therefore lead to superficiality. Long problems need to be studied in advance of the tutorial group, which not only requires considerable organization by the students but also takes away some of the 'freshness' of the problem by the time the tutorial group meets.

One of the causes of long problems is an inappropriate response by planners to external pressures. For example, the faculty may consider that the medical course pays insufficient attention to old people who need wheelchairs, so old ladies in wheelchairs start to appear in problems even though they are quite irrelevant to the problems.

The problem should be easy to read

The vocabulary and readability level should be pitched at the students' ability to comprehend.

The problem should not contain hidden meanings

Sometimes the key to a problem is some hidden agenda on the part of the designer. This is not helpful. Consider the following:

Does one need a paediatric stethoscope for children, or is an adult stethoscope sufficient?

At clinic, a sensible 15-year-old asthmatic girl and her parents reported that she is fine and free from symptoms. There are no abnormalities on listening to her chest. Despite this, the paediatrician insists on a peak flow measurement.

In casualty, a three-year-old girl arrives with a severe attack of asthma. She is very short of breath. The SHO is surprised to find hardly any wheezing at all when she listens to the chest. Four hours later, having progressively worsened, the child collapses and requires artificial ventilation.

A seven-year-old boy with cystic fibrosis is brought to the doctor with new symptoms; a severe cough, fever, and green sputum. On examination the child has a pyrexia, an obvious cough, there is early finger clubbing, but there are no added sounds to be heard on auscultation of the chest. A chest radiograph shows scattered changes; some suggest new infection, others look like more chronic changes. Sputum cultures grow Staphylococcus aureus and Haemophilus influenzae. There is rapid improvement after treatment with intravenous antibiotics.

A 14-year-old boy with asthma says he is symptom-free and never needs his inhalers. His chest is clear to auscultation. His peak flow is only 56% of his best ever figure.

A five-week-old baby presents with a two-day history of coughing, wheezing and difficulty in feeding. The respiratory rate is raised and, on listening to the chest, one hears showers of crepitations all over the chest.

The first four cases are meant to be illustrations of the point that auscultation may be insufficient to detect or diagnose important respiratory disease in childhood. The final case is there to throw the students 'off the scent' with the opposite message, namely that hearing crepitations points to a specific diagnosis (bronchiolitis). The designer of the problem hopes that the students, instead of just looking at these five cases individually, will realize the hidden meaning. To make sure the planner's mission does not fail, the tutors' notes prompt the tutor to ask the students what these cases have in common. The drawback to this strategy is that it risks the students trying to work out the hidden agenda every time they see a case, thereby treating cases as artificial exercises rather than real life problems. The game '20 questions' in which one is allowed 20 questions in order to guess the identity of a word or phrase is great fun, but problems should not lead to students spending time trying to guess what the problem designers had in mind.

PROBLEMS ARE DYNAMIC AND MUST EVOLVE

It is impossible to get the design of a problem right on a first attempt. One would need second sight to know how different groups of students respond to a problem. If at all possible, new problems should be test-run on a group of students, to see what difficulties are encountered, and to see what learning objectives are generated.

A vital role for the tutor is to feed back the difficulties and outcomes (learning objectives) to the planners and problem design group, so that problems can be amended. This is a continuous process. As a course continues to evolve, and the knowledge that students bring changes, problems need to be continually altered and refashioned.

The problem of the 4-year-old child with a rapidly fatal illness (worked example 2, chapter 2) can be taken as an example. The child was given an injection of benzylpenicillin, but died soon after. When this problem was given to fourth year medical students, a number of them considered the possibility that the child had died of an anaphylactic (severe allergy) reaction to penicillin. The planning team might well have found this helpful, for allergic reactions to drugs are a common and important problem. If the topic was felt to be an unhelpful diversion, then possible strategies are to:

- re-word the problem, taking out the name and dose of the antibiotic, or taking out the antibiotic treatment altogether
- instruct the tutors to assist by asking how an anaphylactic reaction could explain the purpuric rash, as a way of helping the students to see that an allergic reaction to antibiotics is an unlikely cause of the child's fatal illness.

39

Another example of the need to re-write a problem follows:

> *Learning objectives: causes of vomiting in an infant; the phenomenon of switching milk formulae*
>
> **Vomiting in a five-week-old baby**
>
> *The parents of Mary Johnson, a five-week-old baby girl, report that she has been vomiting feeds. She usually vomits shortly after the end of a feed, but sometimes vomits during a feed. She was born at term and formula-fed, and the vomiting started when she was about three-to-four days-old. She was initially fed on SMA White Cap but, when Mary was two and a half-weeks-old, the health visitor suggested changing the feed to Cow and Gate Premium because of the vomiting. This change was no help so, at the age of three and a half-weeks, the health visitor suggested changing to Isomil, but again this was no help. For the last week, the vomiting has increased, and Mary's general practitioner has, therefore, referred her to hospital.*
>
> *What is the likely explanation/cause for the child's symptoms, and how does the cause(s) result in vomiting?*

Two difficulties that occurred when this problem was used are shown below, along with the solution.

Issue 1. When given to fourth-year medical students, this problem caused them to focus heavily on the difference between the three types of feed, a discussion which was hampered by a lack of knowledge of the composition of these formulae.

Issue 2. By virtue of the history, the child does not have pyloric stenosis, but one aim of the case was to allow the students to sift through the pros and cons of this common diagnostic problem. The female sex of the child diminished discussion about pyloric stenosis (which is more common in boys) as a possible cause of the symptoms.

Outcome: The child's name was changed from Mary to Mark. The proprietary names of the milk formulae were replaced by the generic terms whey-based milk formula, casein-based milk formula and soya-based milk formula.

If problems in a problem-based learning course are not constantly evolving and being subject to alteration, then it is likely that insufficient attention is being paid to problem design.

EVALUATING THE QUALITY OF THE PROBLEMS IN A CURRICULUM

The quality of the problems in a curriculum has a profound effect on student learning. Evaluative information about different aspects of the problems is needed to improve the problems. There are three main types of information.

1. Students' perceptions

Students' perceptions about the quality of problems can be obtained from student evaluation instruments [14].

2. Problem effectiveness

Problem effectiveness is defined as the degree of correspondence between student-generated learning issues and pre-set faculty objectives [16].

Consider the following problem, which comes from the second year of the medical curriculum in Maastricht [17].

A tall girl

During the past few years, Ellen has grown tall very quickly. She has always been a tall girl, but at the age of 11 years and a height of five feet four inches, she stands head and shoulders above her age group. People always take her to be older, which sometimes becomes wearisome. What will become of her? She still has not reached the age of puberty.

When designing this problem, the planners had five learning objectives in mind:

- what are the normal rates of child growth?
- what are the normal stages in secondary sexual characteristics?
- which endocrine control processes influence growth?
- what are the psychological effects of being significantly taller than others in ones age group?
- what diagnostic procedures are available to predict ultimate height?

When given the problem, one tutorial group generated five learning issues, but they were not the same five as above. They omitted to consider the psychological effects of being tall, but they generated an issue that did not correspond to what the faculty had in mind, namely the type of treatment available to control excessive growth.

The results of a study by Dolmans [17] showed that an average of 64% of the faculty learning objectives were actually generated as learning issues by the students. On average, 15% of the faculty objectives were not identified by the students and these were either related to other curricular activities (such as skills training sessions), were too broadly defined (requiring an extensive search of the literature), or were related to psychology and sociology. The study also showed that 6% of the student-generated learning issues did not correspond to any of the pre-set faculty objectives. However, of these unexpected learning issues, almost a half were relevant to the objectives of the curriculum.

When newly designed problems are implemented, student-generated learning issues can provide useful information about problem effectiveness and suggestions on how problems might be improved.

3. Coverage of course content

Student-generated learning issues only reflect what students *plan* to study but not what they *actually* study. Assessing the latter and comparing it with the intended content provides information about course content coverage. This information can be obtained from questionnaires requiring students to rate the content studied, the time spent on studying the content and the degree to which students master this content [14].

5 TUTORIAL GROUPS AND PARTICIPANT ROLES: PROBLEMS AND SOLUTIONS

ANATOMY OF A TUTORIAL GROUP

A problem-based learning tutorial group consists of:

(a) a group chairperson
(b) a scribe
(c) other students/learners
(d) a tutor.

The roles of individuals are described in this chapter. A good group size (discussed further in chapter 2) is eight to 10 students. If the group is much larger it is impossible for all individuals to participate adequately. If the group is much smaller then there will be too little of an important ingredient, the prior knowledge of the group.

Rotating the chairperson and scribe roles

The roles of the chairperson and scribe should be rotated through the whole tutorial group. These skills, which should be acquired by all students, take time and practice to master.

Regrouping of students

Students should stay within a single tutorial group for a block, module or semester, perhaps seven to 14 weeks, but then the tutorial groups should be split and regrouped.

ATTENDANCE OF STUDENTS AND TUTOR

Compulsory attendance at tutorials for students sits uncomfortably with the principles of adult learning. The problem is that a key ingredient of problem-based learning is the input from fellow students, and if only three students out of a group of eight attends then the three who have come are seriously disadvantaged.

A group is similarly disadvantaged by the absence of a tutor, so it is essential that the tutor attends all tutorial group meetings.

DURATION OF TUTORIAL

A tutorial group may spend one to one and a half hours on a new problem plus one to one and a half hours discussing a previous problem. Course organizers and tutors should not expect three hours of high-class interactive discussion without a short break and the availability of coffee or tea.

TUTORIAL GROUPS AND ROLES

Every member of the group contributes to the process in a different way: by talking or being silent, by making jokes or being serious, by making or not making proposals, or by discussing personal experiences. The chairperson, the scribe, the group members and the tutor all have specific roles that facilitate and assist the tutorial group to function as a whole.

Students unfamiliar with problem-based learning cannot be expected to miraculously acquire the necessary skills as soon as they join a small problem-based learning group. In the initial tutorials, the tutor may have to guide and direct the chairperson, scribe and the students carefully through each step of the tutorial process, their reasoning, their learning needs and in identifying learning resources. Thus, the tutor *models* and demonstrates the behaviours and the process required to work on the problem. As students become adept at the process, the tutor *coaches* and only interjects if the students miss a step in the process, stray from the problem or are stuck or confused. With time, students mature and the level of support from the tutor is reduced. Where problem-based learning is used in the clinical part of the curriculum, the tutor has additional roles (discussed in step 8, chapter 2).

BEHAVIOUR OF THE GROUP WILL CHANGE WITH TIME

Tutorial groups working together tend to progress through four phases. An awareness of these phases helps tutors and students to understand the group's progress and not to be distressed by the inevitable group dysfunctions that occur even in the best of groups with the best of tutors.

(a) Forming

At the outset, group members are on their best behaviour, courteous, friendly and accommodating. Each member holds back any irritations and strong personal opinions.

(b) Storming

After a variable period of time, usually a few weeks, group members are no longer strangers. As they struggle to establish their roles, the individual differences or frustrations about the group's activities surface in a variety of ways: arguments, withdrawal from the group, attempts to dominate, expressions of discomfort.

(c) Norming

Interpersonal issues are resolved and the group arrives at an understanding of how to behave.

(d) Performing

The group members work together productively on the task.

These phases underline the fact that it is inappropriate to have tutorial groups function for less than six to eight weeks. In a shorter period students may never really get comfortable with the small group learning process or with each other, and may never reap the rewards of the performing phase.

Each group is an 'organism' with quite distinct behaviour. No two groups are the same.

ROLE OF THE PROBLEM-BASED LEARNING TUTORIAL GROUP

Key steps in the process

The primary role of the problem-based learning tutorial group is to study the problem systematically, using steps such as 'the seven jump' or 'the eight step' discussion process (discussed in chapter 2). The advantage of a stepped process is to remind students to stop and think reflectively about each learning situation prior to proceeding with the discussion. The purpose of the group discussion is to help students recall what they already know about the issues presented in the problem, to expose their thoughts and beliefs, to exchange, confront and question different views, to clarify their own thinking, to organize ideas within structured networks, to connect main ideas to one another and to their prior knowledge, to hypothesize, to make inferences and eliminate the various alternatives, to raise questions and, finally, to see the need to gather more information. The role of the group is facilitated by a cooperative (as opposed to a competitive) context, and by skills in reading, communicating and thinking.

Reading the problem

Reading the problem starts off the tutorial and is a skill in itself. When reading, students should recognize main ideas and supporting information and be able to differentiate them. A helpful way is to mark the text by underlining main ideas and circling supporting details. This also helps concentrate on what is being read and prevents the mind from wandering to other things.

Communication skills

Communication skills include listening, speaking (questioning, explaining, responding, sharing information, giving and accepting criticism), perspective-taking (exploring another person's thinking and affect, including role play), respecting the views of others and interacting sensitively and humanely.

Listening is a neglected communication skill and hearing does not necessarily imply listening. To be active listeners students should:

- pay attention to the ideas that arise from the discussion (by asking, 'Is this important? Why and how is it important?')
- respond nonverbally by nodding, smiling or frowning
- respond by asking questions or requesting explanations
- make notes.

Note-taking

Note-taking helps listening by providing a logical organization to what is being heard. It is very difficult to listen to and remember disorganized, unrelated bits of information. Although students may make individual notes for themselves, the secretary has the important role of note-taking for the group as a whole.

Speaking

Speaking, instead of just looking and listening, increases involvement in learning. All students should have the opportunity to speak, express their ideas and to contribute to the group's activities. Group members must learn to give each other constructive comments rather than ones which embarrass or intimidate. Constructive comments help to prevent shy students from withdrawing from the group.

Thinking

Thinking will vary with the problem and might include: deliberating or reflecting on the problem; analysing and evaluating evidence and reviewing what is known; creating hypotheses; making decisions about what observations, questions or probes need to be made; appraising, questioning and judging information obtained from inquiry; seeing new relationships, synthesizing, speculating, arguing rationally; pondering about other sources of information; reflecting on what has been learned, what it all may mean and what needs to be done next; transferring skills to new contexts and problem-solving. During the stage of brain-storming, group members 'storm' a problem with ideas. One key to brain-storming is that no criticism is allowed of contributions. As any idea, no matter how wild, is accepted, brain-storming is highly creative and can lead to unexpected avenues of exploration. Brain-storming is followed by the generation of hypotheses, which must of course be exposed to careful evaluation.

ROLE OF THE CHAIRPERSON

Successfully leading a group discussion requires group management skills. These skills are related to (i) the group process, (ii) the logical structure of the discussion and (iii) the content of the discussion. Like many skills, acquiring the skills of leading a group discussion requires practice with feedback. The following are suggestions to help those new to the task.

- Investigate who the group members are. Preliminary introductions help members of a new group to get to know each other.
- Make agreements with group members about the procedure of the discussion: how the problem will be discussed, how the time allotted for the discussion will be spent, how decisions will be made. Make evaluative comments during and at the end of the discussion by asking, 'Does everyone agree with what we are doing and the way this is done?' or 'Is everyone satisfied with this procedure?'
- Introduce the problem for discussion. Ensure that the group members are interested in the problem. If they are not, it may be that they do not feel it is relevant, and this will merit its own short discussion. Keep the introduction

47

neutral, and refrain from expressing opinions as this can influence the opinions of others and dominate the discussion.

- If silent reading of the problem is the preference of the group, then give group members time to read the problem.

- Invite participation from all group members. This can be done verbally ('what do you think?') and nonverbally (chairperson looks at John).

- Summarize or encourage another group member to do so regularly. Ask a group member to paraphrase or restate the response given by another. Summarizing and paraphrasing not only demands constant attention from all group members, but also draws together the key points, unresolved issues and important links. When expressed in an individual's own words and interrogatively, they help group members to concentrate on what is said and whether or not it is correct. Summarizing and paraphrasing strengthens comprehension, promotes deeper understanding and stimulates thoughts and opinions for further discussion.

- When thoughts and opinions are not clearly formulated, it is important to elaborate. For example:

Chairperson: *'John. I'm not quite sure I follow. Why is it that too small a hole in the teat can cause babies to vomit. I don't see why it should. Could you just explain that again in a little more detail?'*

Susan: *'Surely you've got it wrong. It's too large a hole in the teat that causes vomiting. The milk comes so fast that the baby vomits.'*

Chairperson: *'But why should drinking fast make a baby vomit? If I quickly down a few pints, I don't vomit.'*

John: *'The books say that too small a hole in the teat can cause vomiting. But I must admit, now that you mention it, that I can't explain it. Maybe the books are wrong.'*

Jenny: *'I didn't understand this either. I asked Sister Heath about it and she said that what happens is that, when the hole is too small, the baby cannot get much milk and keeps swallowing air. The little milk that is obtained comes back when the air is regurgitated, and the parents complain the baby is vomiting. Sister said that one clue to this is the parents reporting that the baby takes 45–60 minutes to feed; the baby is spending much of that time swallowing air.'*

Jeremy: *'Why do teats come with different sized holes? What are the different sizes?'*

Elaborating helps to keep the discussion on track, to deepen understanding and to stimulate further discussion.

- Stimulate the group to discuss the problem from different angles.
- Set an example that facilitates the group process. By expressing his/her own thoughts and feelings, the group leader can dispel inhibitions that group members might have about contributing their own thoughts and feelings.
- Give process observations to make group members aware about what is happening in the group. For example, group members may be talking to the chairperson rather than with each other. Thank group members for helpful contributions. Although all irrelevant remarks are not likely to interrupt a coherent discussion, those that might throw the group off track must be recognized in a manner that is not embarrassing to the speaker.
- Reformulate the subject concretely mentioning common and any possible opposing views. Check with the group whether or not the reformulation is indeed a reflection of the discussion. After reformulating, make a proposal about how to continue the discussion.
- Bring the discussion to a conclusion. Make decisions about learning goals with the group members. Seek consensus and check that all group members agree with the learning goals.
- Help the group work within the time allotted for the tutorial.

All this may seem a bit overpowering for new students leading groups for the first time. It does all get easier with practice. Leadership is itself a learning process. For more experienced students or graduate students who are well accustomed to working in groups, there may be little or no need for a chairperson.

ROLE OF THE SCRIBE

The scribe has the important role of note-taking, usually using a flip-chart, overhead transparency or white/black board. Organized notes help the group to identify important ideas and provide a record that facilitates learning and remembering. The following steps help good note-taking.

- Listen carefully to the discussion. If uncertain, ask the group what was said and whether or not it should be written down.
- Note down ideas and concepts no matter how trivial or far-fetched they might seem, but do not attempt to write down every word that is said.

49

- Organize the notes by categorizing concepts. For example, in a two-day-old infant with jaundice, one would categorize this as either being conjugated or unconjugated hyperbilirubinaemia. The most important part of note-taking is to present the information as a whole with all its relationships and interconnected parts. Organizing concepts requires analyses rather than merely memorizing, and helps students to understand what they are studying. Organized notes are also easier to remember.
- Review the notes with group members to check that they are representative of the group's thoughts and concepts.
- Use abbreviations that other group members are familiar with.
- Do not forget that the scribe is still a contributing member of the group! It is difficult to do well both the task of scribe and participate actively in the discussion. If the scribe becomes involved with the discussion as much as other group members, the scribing may be poor. If the scribe does not participate and simply writes things down mechanically, he or she will lose out. The trick is for the scribe to follow the discussion by mentally leading it, which will enable the scribe to make some contributions while actively thinking about the problem.
- Leave space so that information may be added later. One way is to take notes of main ideas on the left side of the flip-chart or board, leaving the right side blank for adding supporting details, comments, questions, examples or restated thoughts.
- Highlight important concepts, for example by underlining or the use of capital letters.
- Do not misuse the position of standing near the flip-chart and of holding the pen by being authoritarian and judgemental. Do not write down your own contributions but selectively ignore contributions of others!
- Groups can be well controlled by a good scribe. For example, 'I need to know what you are saying to put it on the flip-chart' is a useful and helpful way of guiding and focusing thought.

ROLE OF THE TUTOR

Although tutoring in problem-based learning is quite different from lecturing, it does not amount to thoughtless silence! Effective tutoring involves a constellation of skills, attitudes and knowledge that reflects the needs of tutorial groups for guidance in both task accomplishment and maintenance of productive working relationships. Above all, it requires intense concentration.

1. Modelling behaviours that students will adopt

The tutor should model behaviours that keep the learning process moving and ensure that no step of the learning process is neglected.

2. Promoting student direction and facilitating group interactions

Arrange seating

Seating affects patterns of interaction [18]. Interactions between students are most likely to occur when their seating is arranged so that they face each other around a table (compare the interactions around a dinner table with those in a series of rows of seats in an auditorium). The tutor should be seated with the students, and in a way that does not set the tutor apart from the students (for example sitting behind the students, or in some focal point eg at the head of a table). Interactions are further increased by varying the seating pattern in each tutorial: talkative students may be inhibited if seated close to the tutor or chairperson, and shy students are more likely to make contributions if seated opposite the tutor or chairperson.

Create a 'safe' environment

Fear of the unknown and feeling threatened or intimidated deter students from contributing. It is therefore important to clarify expectations to create a safe environment and allay anxieties. This allows students to take risks, to ask questions that might seem trivial and to try out ideas which may be wrong without being humiliated or ridiculed. The tutor should avoid expressing opinions concerning the correctness or quality of students' contributions and should avoid displaying favouritism. The tutor must also respect students and be patient while they struggle with new ideas.

Facilitate interpersonal relationships

The tutor must be aware of the interpersonal dynamics at work in the group and have skills in managing interpersonal conflict. This is discussed later in the chapter under the heading 'Problems of Interpersonal Dynamics'.

Praise and feedback

Praise (at the end of the tutorial session) when a group of students makes a good point, a valid inference or adopt a creative approach to the problem shows that

51

helpful contributions are valued and encourages rich interactions. Thanking the group for its contributions and pointing out what has been achieved is healthy for group morale and group functioning.

Avoid dominating the discussion

To facilitate student interactions the tutor must avoid being the focus of any discussions. Different strategies can be used to deflect attention from the tutor. When a student addresses the tutor with a statement or question, the tutor can say, 'Who has some thoughts about this comment (or question)?' or can look at another student for a response. Non-participating students may be drawn into the discussion by questions aimed directly at them (which must be carried out with care, as it can be potentially intimidating). A tutor intervening with the intention to help can easily dominate a discussion by asking narrowly focused questions, or not giving students enough time to think and respond, or giving extended answers to students' questions. The solution to this is to ask probing questions that open up rather than close down a discussion, and to replace offering complete answers that end the discussion with making brief statements that moves thinking forward.

3. Guiding the group's learning

Let students explore ideas

Students must be allowed to develop and explore ideas during the discussion. They should not be prevented from making mistakes. The tutor should guide the students' thinking through appropriate questions until they naturally and automatically develop the habit of challenging each other with similar questions. In this way, deliberate and reflective thinking becomes a group habit through practice.

Intervene appropriately

Tutors should listen attentively, be sensitive to students' needs, judge the best moment to intervene and provide information when it is appropriate to do so. Any intervention should enhance the discussion and learning rather than exert control. Intervention may be needed to encourage students expressing different views, challenge thinking, stop digression, refocus the discussion, synthesize perspectives, highlight critical points or subtly raise additional points to be considered.

Guide covertly

The guidance should be covert so that it is not apparent to the students and they continue to feel they are in charge (in control) of the learning process.

For example, ask, 'Are there other possibilities you might not have thought of?' if students have not entertained the correct hypothesis as to the underlying mechanism for a problem. Or, 'Let's stop and review our hypotheses again.' if a new finding requires new hypotheses.

This guidance should be given both when students' opinions or statements are correct as well as incorrect, to avoid the tutor's questions turning into a signal that the students are on the wrong track. Students are exquisitely sensitive to the behaviour of the tutor and will be watching the tutor out of the corners of their eyes. The slightest signals can alter the course of the discussion. One of the most common errors of tutors is to stall discussion completely by being too heavy-handed.

Probe and challenge students' thinking

The tutor should probe and challenge students' thinking and understanding with questions [18].

Examples of probing and challenging questions

'Does that always apply?'
'Why do you want to know that?'
'How is that relevant?'
'Can you tell us what you mean?'
'Can you give us an example?'
'Is there an alternative viewpoint?'
'How do you know that is true?'
'How reliable is the evidence?'
'How accurate is your description?'
'Are you sure you're right?'
'Are you comfortable with that explanation?'
'You say it is $\underline{x}$, which particular kind of $\underline{x}$?'
'What is the underlying principle?'
'In what situation would this rule break down?'
'What distinguishes the two cases?'

Controversy, raised by challenging students' ideas, opinions and conclusions, can trigger the cycle of learning by arousing feelings of uncertainty, conceptual conflict, curiosity and intrinsic motivation. The tutor's questions should make students aware of what questions they should be asking themselves as they tackle the problem. They should also help students to understand the problem from their concepts of basic science principles, or pathophysiology, or other disciplines such as humanities or social sciences. They should always be reinforcing and not undermining.

Be clear about course objectives

Tutors must be clear about the objectives of the course, the principles that students are expected to master and need to ensure that students meet important curricular objectives with their problems. They must be familiar with the curriculum and be aware of students' level of prior knowledge. Tutors also have a responsibility to ensure that students recognize any doubts they may have about the correctness or sufficiency of their knowledge and that they note this as a learning objective.

Acknowledge ignorance

It is impossible for any tutor to be familiar with the wide variety of concepts (including basic science, psychosocial and ethical) included in multidisciplinary tutorial problems. A tutor admitting ignorance and willingly participating in learning sets an example to students that there is no limit to learning.

4. Motivating students to learn

Motivation enhances learning and retention. The tutor must motivate students by arousing their interest in the problem, for example challenging their thoughts, helping them to see the relevance of the problem or helping them appreciate what they will need to learn.

5. Monitoring the progress of each student in the group

The final (or block or semester) examination is not the time to find out about a poorly performing student: by then it is far too late. Monitoring the progress of each student in the group is an important tutor role. Well before a student falls too far behind to catch up and continued learning is progressively more difficult, the tutor should identify learning difficulties, difficulties in understanding information and concepts, or problems in finding appropriate information through self-directed study, in order to provide timely and appropriate help. Thus, the tutor may have to challenge the student gently in an area in which he or she is suspected to have difficulty.

6. Monitoring attendance

In most problem-based learning courses, attendance at the tutorials is compulsory, and the tutor has a role in reporting absences.

7. Providing feedback to management/planning group

As discussed in chapter 4 on problem design, it is important that the tutor provides feedback to the management group or course planners about (a) any organizational problems, and (b) the performance of individual problems, which may need to be amended, re-written or scrapped altogether.

8. Helping students to identify learning resources

The course module handbook (discussed at the end of this chapter) should give some useful suggestions for learning resources, but the tutor will be well placed to guide students who are considering other types of learning resource. For example, in the clinical part of the curriculum, the students might tackle a problem that includes the topic of cervical screening. The students (or the tutor) might come up with the idea of going to visit a laboratory that does cervical cytology, to see how it is done. The tutor should be able to give some practical guidance, saving fruitless telephone calls and wasted trips.

With an increasing emphasis on using the community as a resource, a tutor with his or her local knowledge can be invaluable either by pointing students to think of community resources (if this has not crossed their mind) or to suggest which types of resource might be worth exploring.

Tutors can also help students to identify themselves as learning resources. For example, in a problem in which it appears that the patient has cancer of the cervix, the students (in the clinical curriculum) might not consider a practical issue such as the need for urgency in referring a patient to hospital. A good way to bring this out, and one that will also introduce students to the whole process of hospital referral, is to suggest that the students draft a general practitioner's letter of referral. Students usually pick up the issue of urgency when they discuss the appropriate wording, but if they do not the tutor can suggest they discuss how letters of referral are processed when they reach the hospital. Note that the guidance is indirect; the tutor never need direct the group by asking bluntly 'how urgent is this referral?'.

PROBLEMS IN THE WAY STUDENTS TACKLE A PROBLEM-BASED LEARNING TASK

Students come to university with a range of learning strategies acquired from school experience as well as from other life experiences. Problems in the way that students

55

tackle a problem-based learning task are related to poor learning strategies, for example strategies that permit them to avoid learning new information by classifying it as 'already known'. These strategies, and how the problems might be overcome, are described briefly in this section.

1. Failing to question the correctness of prior knowledge

Students who use this strategy recall prior knowledge and link it with new information. However, they fail to question the *correctness* of their prior knowledge, which may be incomplete or incorrect, and they therefore do not modify their prior knowledge. Students may even ignore or distort new information in the problem to make it 'fit' with their existing knowledge.

Given that much prior knowledge consists of naive beliefs and uncontrolled everyday experiences, significant changes need to be made to students' naive knowledge structures for them to understand and remember new concepts appropriately. To do this, tutors need to be able to identify errors in what students know and to help students see that their own existing concepts are in conflict with scientific data, that their notions are inadequate, incomplete or inconsistent, and that a scientific explanation provides a more convincing and powerful alternative to their own notions. This can be done through individual questioning or presenting an 'exposing' situation that invites students' comments and confrontation of each others' ideas.

2. Failing to recognize new information as 'unknown' or 'new', assuming there is nothing new to learn

This is not quite the same as the preceding problem. Students who exhibit this strategy will report knowing everything there is to know about the content of a problem, and they may do so even before they have read the problem. Instead of using the information in the problem to recall and reflect on what is known and to answer questions, students think the information is simply repetitious. The task for the tutor is to question and challenge the students' 'knowledge'.

3. Overfocusing on text vocabulary

Students who exhibit this strategy view learning as vocabulary acquisition. They isolate new words and phrases in the problem and, having done so, feel they comprehend the problem. The words and phrases are likely to be taken out of context and are not put into the context of the students' own experiences. A series of thoughtfully designed open-ended questions from the tutor may encourage students to see that their task is not simply to decode new words but to use prior knowledge about word sequence, word meaning and the relevance of the context to understand the information in the problem.

4. Overfocusing on unrelated facts

Students who exhibit this strategy see learning as mere fact acquisition. Students simply add facts to memory as isolated bits of information unrelated to other ideas. They can recall facts but can neither link them to relevant concepts nor apply them to appropriate situations. Given that all students have some relevant knowledge to which new facts can be related, tutors can facilitate learning by having students recall the relevant knowledge, describe examples from their experiences, or use the context of the new information to form conceptual bridges between what they already know and what they are learning.

5. Overfocusing on one aspect

Students may focus on just one detail of the problem that is most appealing to them. This will be studied in depth but, probably due to lack of time, all other important aspects of the problem are neglected. Provided the problem is adequately designed, the tutor can help by questioning students about the other aspects and in a manner that reveals their importance.

6. Superficiality of discussion

There is a tendency for discussions to remain superficial, thus compromising the quality and creativity of students' conclusions and their depth of understanding. Students may use terms and concepts without having to dig to deeper levels to answer why, what, where and when. The tutor has to probe for deeper and fuller explanations and for descriptions of phenomena at a more basic level. Hypothesizing is a useful way of deepening the discussion.

7. Adopting the role of the physician

Confronted with patients' problems, students tend to adopt the role of physician. They are anxious to solve the problem of the patient, to establish the diagnosis and subsequently focus their study activities on the treatment of that particular disease. In doing so, they are likely to avoid studying the aetiology of the disease and understanding the clinical features in terms of underlying basic mechanisms. They may also forget to look at a problem from the patient's point of view. For example, in a problem about routine ante-natal care and what happens at the 'booking clinic' (the first visit to the hospital ante-natal clinic), students usually have no idea what information should be provided. However if they are encouraged to imagine that they are the expecting-mother or her partner, and asked to think of what sort of problems they would be worried about, groups will be full of ideas.

PROBLEMS OF INTERPERSONAL DYNAMICS

Interpersonal problems may arise in any tutorial group and can inhibit its effectiveness. They do not surface until the group members have begun to get to know one another. Symptoms of disharmony or ineffectiveness [19,20] in the group include:

- lack of progress because the group cannot agree on where to go with the problem or spend a long time on cyclic or trivial discussions
- reluctance by good students to share or pool information because they feel they are 'carrying' lazy or weak students
- silence
- late arrival
- sarcasm
- lack of individual productivity
- lack of spontaneity
- arguments in place of relaxed discussions
- students taking sides on an issue
- covert, manipulative contests between students
- expressions of dissatisfaction with learning
- attempts by students to take over.

An awareness that these problems may surface at any time is a key to managing these problems. The earlier they are recognized, the more effectively and promptly they can be handled.

The tutor should not take on a parental or fully responsible role in dealing with these interpersonal problems. This will make the students dependent on the tutor, who is then expected to solve the problem. Students must themselves learn to deal with interpersonal dynamics as they will inevitably have to do so in their professional careers.

If possible, it is helpful to let the problem go long enough for a group member to recognize it and express concern. The tutor may have to intervene early by saying, 'We aren't making progress. What do you suppose is going on?' and 'What shall we do about it?'

If the ensuing discussions cannot resolve the problem, then the group has to talk about their behaviours and feelings and design a way to manage them. The group can get together before a session, after a session or one evening for an open-ended discussion about its interpersonal problem. It should be clear to the group members that they do not have to like each other, but they do have to learn to work together effectively.

CONTINUING STAFF DEVELOPMENT FOR TUTORS

One would not expect someone to become a problem-based learning tutor without attending one or more staff development sessions for people intending to take on this role. Once initial training has been received, there is a need for more advanced training, including the facility to train on topics such as dealing with difficult individuals or groups (using role playing students or staff), and giving feedback to students. Although major problems with tutor behaviour should be picked up as the result of feedback from students to faculty, a continuing programme of staff development is part of quality management in problem-based learning.

Full details of staff development are outside the scope of this book. However, a brief outline of one possible approach to a one-day training programme 'Introduction to Problem-based Learning' for staff who wish to become problem-based learning tutors is given in Table 1. A number of variations on this programme are possible. For example, one strategy is to video a group of students working through steps 1–5, a few days before the training day, and then watch them in action performing steps 7 (and 8 if dealing with the clinical curriculum). It must be emphasized that the programme in Table 1 is more of an 'introduction to problem-based learning' than 'tutor training' and, for the latter one, would certainly want to include the topic of dealing with problem situations in tutorials — useful tools here include video clips of problem and participants taking the role of specific types of difficult behaviour, enabling the tutors in training to practise dealing with these difficulties.

59

TABLE 1 BRIEF OUTLINE OF A ONE-DAY STAFF DEVELOPMENT PROGRAMME FOR STAFF WHO WISH TO BECOME PROBLEM-BASED LEARNING TUTORS

9.30–9.50	All participants: Introduction to problem-based learning and the 7- or 8-step process.
9.50–10.20	Break into groups of eight to 10, one experienced problem-based learning tutor per group. Get group to apply steps 1 to 5 to a non-medical problem suitable for all participants (eg thunderclap problem — see page 31). There is unlikely to be sufficient time for the group to complete all 5 steps, but they are likely to experience the fascination and fun of the process.
10.20–10.50	All participants: Discussion of the process that has taken place, if possible with some explanation of how the 7 or 8 steps fit with what we know about how adults learn.
10.50–11.10	Coffee break
11.10–11.25	All participants: Introduction to problem design.
11.25–12.10	Break into groups. Chosing a topic that will be familiar to the remaining groups (i) select three to five learning objectives and (ii) write an interesting short paper problem designed to lead students to select similar learning objectives.
12.10–13.00	Groups exchange problems. Each group tackles a problem, using the first 5 steps of the process, the experienced tutors ensuring that each group produces a list of learning objectives.
13.00–13.45	Lunch
13.45–14.30	All participants: Comparison of, for example, group A's intended learning objectives vs learning objectives produced when group A's problem studied by group B. Discussion and analysis of problems to identify items that would need altering for future use of the problem.
14.30–15.00	All participants: Introduction to tutor role.
15.00–15.30	Break into groups. (a) role play — dealing with dysfunctional or problem individuals: members of group scripted to behave or misbehave in a particular manner while tackling a problem. One member of group takes tutor role.
15.30–15.50	Tea break
15.50–16.20	Stay in groups. (b) working with students — one member of group acts as tutor to group of problem-based learning medical students, rest of group observing.
16.20–17.00	All participants and students: Discussion of tutor role and how to cope with problems.

By introducing problem-based learning into a course, one is effectively training students to be a generation ahead of the staff. One implication of this is that, once one has started to implement problem-based learning, students who are familiar with the technique are potentially an invaluable resource in staff development.

COURSE MODULE HANDBOOK FOR STUDENTS

Students will need a handbook for each module of a problem-based learning course.

60

The handbook should provide:

- basic information about the module
- the text of all written problems and some information about other types of trigger material
- an opportunity for students to plan their learning. One example would be making a note of learning objectives for which there was insufficient time available
- several opportunities for reflection (for example keeping a note of issues or patients seen, with a brief note of ones thoughts, experiences and plans for the future)
- several opportunities for self-assessment (discussed in more detail in the next chapter). An illustrative example is given in Figure 1.
- an opportunity to record the experience obtained before qualification
- a list of module objectives in terms of knowledge ('By the end of the module you should understand the social influences on diet and nutrition')
- a description of the learning environment, where the students will be working, names of tutors with a timetable if there is one
- information about type of learning resources and their availability
- details of plans for skills development and a list of skills objectives (for example 'Take a full history of the gastrointestinal system', with an indication of whether or not the skill has been observed or practised and, if so, how many times)
- suggested reading list.

Here is an opportunity to assess yourself. Below is a list of objectives and a grid for you to decide how confident you CURRENTLY feel about them. You should ring an appropriate number from 1 (not at all confident) to 5 (very confident)					
Date of completion					
I understand the structure and function of the cardiovascular system	1	2	3	4	5
I understand the structure and function of the respiratory system	1	2	3	4	5
I understand the structure and function of the haematological system	1	2	3	4	5
I can describe the epidemiology of three major conditions affecting these systems	1	2	3	4	5
I could explain to a patient what hypertension is	1	2	3	4	5
I can take a full history of a problem in the respiratory system	1	2	3	4	5
I can take a full history from a patient with a blood problem	1	2	3	4	5
I can examine the cardiovascular system	1	2	3	4	5
I can examine the respiratory system	1	2	3	4	5
I could give a patient details of the diagnosis of a blood disease	1	2	3	4	5

Figure 1 Example of self-assessment in a module handbook for a first clinical year module entitled 'Heart Lungs and Blood'

COURSE MODULE NOTES FOR TUTOR

These are only for the use of tutors and course managers, and are used in conjunction with the module handbook.

The notes should contain:

- some guidance on conducting problem-based learning tutorial groups (the nature of the guidance will depend on the nature and amount of training that is given to all tutors)
- notes on the problems/trigger material, indicating the intended learning objectives and suggested learning resources. The notes may give specific comments on items in a problem. For example, in a problem about abdominal pain and diarrhoea, the first sentences of the problem might be:

'Jenny Lever, a 19-year-old waitress, went to the hospital casualty complaining of a seven-day history of abdominal pain and diarhhoea. The restaurant where she works has told her that she must not come to work.'

The tutor notes might point out:
— her job implies that she handles food
— attending casualty suggests there is a reason why she might not attend her GP
— not being allowed to go to work: students may wish to consider public health/occupational medicine issues and rules about food handling.

If a tutor is a member of the module planning team, has helped to prepare the problems, is familiar with the learning objectives for each case, and is an expert in the topic, then tutor notes may not be crucial. However on most occasions the tutor will not be in this position, in which case these type of notes are essential.

Notes for tutors should not be given to students. Their use by students would undermine the whole process of problem-based learning.

6 SELF-ASSESSMENT, PEER-ASSESSMENT AND TUTOR ASSESSMENT

The aim of this chapter is to introduce some basic principles. What are the different types of assessment? Are assessments needed in problem-based learning, or should they be avoided altogether? What good and what harm can assessments do? What effect do assessments have on students?

The word assessment is used with a dual meaning, referring to formal assessments (ie examinations) and informal assessments ('how did I do in the tutorial today?').

Assessment is a crucial component of learning. Students cannot realize that they have learned unless they can gauge the extent and depth of learning. Thus, if students are to be involved in their own learning, it is evident that they must be active partners in their own evaluation. They cannot be evaluated by a system that treats them as mere numbers in a bureaucratic game.

TWO MAIN TYPES OF ASSESSMENT

Formative assessment

The aim of formative assessments is to give the student feedback on his or her progress. There are two phases, the assessment itself and the feedback to the student. It should be self-evident, but the prompt availability of feedback is an essential component. We emphasize this because (to our dismay) we are aware of formative assessments in which feedback is either incomplete, delayed for very long periods (for example three to six months), or not given at all. All of these defeat the purpose of the exercise.

In knowledge-based assessments, for example multiple choice questions, feedback can be facilitated by allowing the students to keep the questions, so that they can look up the answers.

In skills-based assessments, such as the objective structured clinical examination (OSCE), feedback can be timetabled in. For example, after a four-minute OSCE station where a student is asked to explain a diagnosis of asthma to the parent of a

63

newly diagnosed child, the next four-minute station can be a feedback station, where the examiner (and the surrogate parent) can give the student immediate feedback.

Summative assessment

The purpose of a summative assessment is to determine whether or not the performance of a student is good enough to allow him or her to proceed to the next part of the course, to graduate, to be licensed to practise or exceptionally to decide if a student should be expelled from a course. In theory, there is no obligation to provide feedback although, in practice, feedback is essential for a student who is to continue on the course.

Combined formative and summative assessment

It is possible to make an assessment both formative and summative, for example by using the assessment to grade while also giving feedback.

Grading of performance

It is possible to grade the performance of students during assessments, and it is possible to reference the result of an individual to the rest of the group (norm referencing) or to some existing standard (criterion referencing).

Honours, distinctions and prizes

Many universities have systems for awarding honours, distinctions and prizes for special performance. A notable exception is McMaster medical school in Canada where, to discourage competition, the final assessment was limited to satisfactory/ provisional satisfactory/unsatisfactory, with no prizes or awards for academic performance [21].

It has been strongly argued [22,23] that rewards such as grades, honours or prizes have a detrimental effect on motivation and run wholly counter to the philosophy of adult learning theory.

THE EFFECT OF ASSESSMENTS ON STUDENTS AND STUDENT LEARNING BEHAVIOUR

Assessments drive student learning [24]. If one gives true/false tests that assess recall of isolated facts in anatomy, students will memorize facts in anatomy. If, on the other hand, one assesses students on their ability to take a history and do a physical examination, they will try to get some clinical teaching and experience. One can devise the most brilliant integrated problem-based learning course in the area of basic medical sciences for first year medical students but, if all they have to do is to pass an examination which tests factual knowledge in anatomy, then that is what they will cram. In other words, the wrong type of assessments can wreck a whole course.

The debate really centres on whether or not this steering effect of assessments is a good or bad thing [25]. What approaches should be taken? The following are some options.

Avoid all assessments

Some believe that the adverse consequences of assessment are so bad that they opt for a strategy that avoids all forms of assessment. The main difficulty with this approach is uncertainty on the part of students, who may have little idea about their own progress, and who may be significantly disadvantaged when finally they are exposed to a formal examination, for example an examination that will license them to practice medicine. Failure to identify students with difficulties makes it impossible to help them.

Avoid targeting the assessment to the curriculum

Some medical schools (including Maastricht, McMaster and Manchester) administer a comprehensive assessment a few times a year to all students; students at all levels take the same test [21,26]. Because the assessment covers the whole field of medicine, students cannot study for the whole test. This encourages students to learn continually and effectively, and not to cram before a test which results in superficial learning.

Use the power of assessment to drive student learning

The third strategy is to deliberately use the assessment to stimulate learning in a particular direction. For example, if it is deemed important that a doctor has the

65

ability to communicate in writing at the level of the person in the street, then it is possible (and done in Manchester) to devise an assessment in which students are instructed to write, using lay terms, a summary and explanation of an article published in a medical journal.

Because assessment drives student learning, it is important that any assessment that does take place focuses on major educational goals.

PRINCIPLES OF ASSESSING STUDENT PERFORMANCE

From the foregoing some basic principles can be distilled. These are listed below.

1. Assessment procedures should be consonant with the aims of the programme.
2. Students must be able to learn from the assessment procedures used.
3. Students must be given an opportunity to display their strengths and not just their weaknesses.
4. Assessment is a shared responsibility. It should, wherever possible, not just be an assessment imposed and controlled by faculty.

SELF-ASSESSMENT AND PEER-ASSESSMENT

If one considers the individual student, he/she may be assessed by himself/herself (self-assessment), by other students in the tutorial group (peer-assessment) or by staff (tutor assessment, examinations).

General principle

In problem-based learning, process and content are inextricably linked. Thus *what* is learned is significantly determined by *how* it is learned. It is therefore important to evaluate both components. Consider the *process* elements first. In the tutorial group it is expected that, when students are presented with a novel problem in the form of a case or a scenario, they will be able to generate issues, organize these into learning tasks, seek appropriate information from a variety of sources, analyse critically the information obtained, synthesize the information into a coherent framework and share the information obtained. They are also expected to facilitate the learning of others, *assess* their own performance as well as their peers on an ongoing basis, and help their peers *assess* their own performances. Since all these elements contribute to effective tutorial performance, it is desirable to evaluate the performance of these elements. This is not easy and there is no foolproof technique. Nevertheless, students benefit greatly from appropriate tutorial evaluation and attempts must be made to set up a 'culture of evaluation'.

Self-assessment

In problem-based learning, students should develop the ability to assess for themselves how effective their processes of learning are. Elements of the assessment of their capacity to learn as a group include collaboration, mutual support, self-direction and a respectful criticism of the ideas offered for analysis of the problem. Because the assessment will help the individual and the group to function more effectively it should ideally be its own reward.

Self-assessment of factual knowledge is restricted to the study of multiple choice questions and textbooks specially written for the purpose.

Long-term aims of self- and peer-assessment

Self and peer-assessment of the learning process have the much more important and long-term aims of developing the skills of communication, cooperation, hypothesis building and analysis, lateral thinking and recognition of uncertainty in available knowledge. These are adult perceptions that the students may take on trust; they embrace them with enthusiasm in the early stages if they see that the group learning process is more enjoyable and gives them more freedom than they have had on other courses. The group may however become dysfunctional if some of its members feel that they are not progressing quickly enough with knowledge acquisition. The formal processes of taking stock of how the group sees itself and of each individual's view of the group are important, even if they lack precision.

ASSESSMENT AND REPORTING BY TUTORS: SHOULD IT HAPPEN?

The main aims of tutors are promoting student direction, facilitating group interaction, guiding the group's learning, and motivating students to learn. One might very well argue that having the tutor monitor student progress and attendance somewhat conflicts with the concept that students are totally independant adults and self-directed learners. In particular there is an anxiety that the 'spy' role of monitoring attendance may set tutors apart from students, thereby undermining the most important roles of the tutor. In an ideal and 'pure adult learning' world, tutors would not monitor attendance or report to faculty on student progress. In practice, because of University work and attendance regulations, and because (in the UK) the payment of student grants depends on attendance, tutors are likely to have to report to the faculty on attendance and performance of individual students. In theory, if one has sufficient resources, one way round the problem is to employ a separate cadre of tutors whose sole role is to visit and observe tutorial groups, reporting on student attendance and student performance (and in addition tutor performance!).

ASSESSMENT BY TUTORS — MANCHESTER MODEL

Assessment is an opportunity for the faculty to reassure students and to suggest actions for improvement, however good the groups (or individual students) feel they are.

An example of one strategy, taken from years 1 and 2 of the Manchester medical curriculum, is given here. Early in a new semester, each student is given an assessment document. The tutors then discuss with their groups the assessment process. The exercise each student is asked to undertake is to review their own and the groups' activities under four headings and to rate their conclusions on a scale from 0 to 8 for each one. The headings are:-

1. Commitment

Consideration here is of motivation, interest and enthusiasm, punctuality, attentiveness and preparation.

2. Interpersonal relationships

The group is asked to reflect on the degree of mutual assistance and support, its sensitivity, and its ability to manage conflict.

3. Group interaction and activity

The relevance of individual contributions, task-sharing, the effectiveness of roles and the development of group roles are listed under this variable.

4. Problem-solving abilities

The group assesses its abilities to define problems, seek solutions and analyse them. It should also review the frequency with which it consults the tutor or gets bogged down in discussion.

There is some guidance on what a good, average or poor student (or group) response might be. This guidance is based not just on theoretical principles but on the experience of the tutors. The group has the assessment document for several weeks before their responses have to be submitted. They will eventually reach a group decision and will do that in consultation with their tutor. The group reflects on its overall performance, whereas its members think about their own contributions and how they may have been affected by their colleagues.

As an additional exercise early in the semester, tutors are required to see each of their students on a one-to-one basis. Students may reveal any misgivings about the course or the way the group functions for them. Members of the group who are quiet or silent during tutorials (or any other students for that matter) can change a tutor's perceptions at this discussion. The students initially assume that the benefit of the whole exercise is the mark obtained. The need to stop and talk with one another, to disagree and then produce a verdict is taken for granted until tutors remind them of the progress they have made from their earliest attempts to work as a group.

In this Manchester model, each student will be credited with the collective group mark, unless an individual student has had unwarranted absences from tutorials, in which case there is a deduction in that individual student's mark. Tutorial groups, particularly those with an unusually high or low score, are visited during one of their sessions by a tutor from another group. The opinion of the visiting tutor is required before the formal assessment process is complete.

A notable exception to this four-part process is an assessment of feedback and evaluation. Figure 1 (overleaf) illustrates how this might be done, using the same rating scale. In this illustration, the areas to consider include regularity of assessments, the process of feedback exchanges, and improvements made as a result of evaluations.

(Ring ONE number)

3 (Poor)	4.5	6 (Competent)	7	8 (Outstanding)
IN THE POOR GROUP		IN THE SATISFACTORY (COMPETENT) GROUP		IN THE OUTSTANDING GROUP
Group evaluations rarely occur		Evaluation sessions happen sometimes		Evaluation sessions are planned frequently
Members never self-evaluate		Members sometimes self-evaluate		Members often self-evaluate
Members show little motivation		Members are keen to improve their functioning as a group		Members are committed to continuous improvement in their functioning
WHEN GIVING FEEDBACK:				
People make general comments		Most comments are specific and concrete		All comments are clearly described and refer to specific behaviours
People make judgements and interpretations		Most comments are descriptive and not judgemental		People never make judgements and always refer to actual behaviour
Comments are not timely		Comments are usually well-timed		Comments are always well-timed
Few members contribute to feedback sessions		Most members contribute to feedback sessions		All members contribute to feedback sessions
Comments are critical and rarely supportive		Most comments are supportive and rarely critical		All comments are supportive and never critical
Comments often start with negative points		Most comments often start positively and finish with negative points		All comments start positively and finish with what could be improved
Clear points for improvement are rarely resolved		Clear points for improvement are usually identified		Specific points for improvement are always identified
Improvement does not occur, and problems continue to happen		Improvement often occurs based on evaluation		Targeted areas always improve after evaluation sessions

Figure I   An assessment instrument — Manchester model — for evaluation and feedback

ASSESSMENT BY STUDENTS — McMASTER MODEL

Usually 15 to 20 minutes are set apart for evaluation and both group and individual performances are evaluated after each tutorial. Students take turns commenting on their own performance as well as that of the group. The process looks reasonable, but is often converted into a mechanical routine where little or no useful evaluation occurs unless a crisis emerges. This is largely because there are no precise or formal guidelines given.

In an effort to introduce some structure into the process, one of us (PKR, in conjunction with students and a colleague) has produced specific forms. These are used at the end of each tutorial. These forms indicate specific categories that are to be considered during evaluation.

The five specific categories to be assessed include:

- Responsibility
- Information
- Communication
- Critical sense
- Self-assessment.

Students are given descriptors that indicate the behaviours that would be exhibited by an outstanding and a poor student in each of those categories (Figure 2). It is important to bracket the range of behaviours so that students can obtain a sense of where they fitted into the spectrum on each day. We have preferred to give descriptors for extreme situations rather than all interim categories. It is emphasized to the students that for the category 'outstanding' a student should perform *consistently* in all categories. Checklists have been avoided to prevent this from becoming a mechanical exercise. For instance, a student who performed all the tasks, but participated actively most of the time and did not really encourage the participation of others would rank him/herself in the B+ or A- category for responsibility.

Each student is given a form (Figure 3) on which they grade their performance at the end of each tutorial using the descriptors provided. They take turns assessing their performance by reading out the grades they have given themselves in each specific category, indicating the reasons why they felt that the grade was justified. The other students and the tutor comment on the self-assessments. If there is a general agreement that the student has accurately assessed himself/herself, a high mark is given for self-assessment. Since the tutor is an essential component, specific forms have been developed to permit the tutors to assess their own performances as well (Figure 4). It is repeatedly stressed that this is formative assessment and every effort should be made for individual students to grade their performances as accurately as possible. These assessments only work if sufficient time is set aside.

71

Categories	Outstanding (A+)	Poor (D)
	the student consistently:	
Responsibility	• completes assigned tasks	• fails to complete assigned tasks
	• participates actively	• participates marginally in tutorials
	• listens to others	• does not listen
	• adds information where appropriate	• confuses others with inappropriate comments
	• encourages participation of others	• does not encourage participation of others
	• does not impede tutorial process by interrupting	• impedes tutorial process by interrupting
	• facilitates learning of others	• does not facilitate the learning of others
Information	• brings in information which is new, relevant, and complements that brought by others	• brings in no new information or provides irrelevant information
	• uses a variety of sources (texts, journals, reviews)	• uses very few sources of information
Communication	• communicates ideas clearly/ concisely	• rambles on or is inaudible
	• ensures that others are not con- fused by information presented	• confuses others
Critical sense	• justifies comments with appropriate references	• fails to justify comments made
	• promotes a deeper understanding of the subject	• fails to promote a deeper understanding of the subject
	• challenges information brought, permitting others to evaluate relevance/significance of their comments	• fails to question/challenge others and thus does not permit them to assess relevance/significance of their comments
Self-assessment	• recognizes strengths and weaknesses	• fails to recognize personal strengths and weaknesses
	• accepts criticism gracefully	• fails to accept constructive criticism gracefully
	• identifies means to correct weaknesses	• becomes defensive and argumentative and does not identify means to correct weaknesses
	• demonstrates effective action to correct weaknesses	• fails to demonstrate effective action to correct weaknesses

Figure 2   Student profile

At intervals, summative assessment occurs using the same categories. Here, however, the emphasis is on peer- rather than on self-assessment. Each student is given a grid indicating the names of the students and the stated categories (Figure 3). The students assess their peers but not themselves on this grid and come prepared for a free and open discussion. At the assessment session, each student's

Course no.: 3A06   Term: I   Student: SJ   Tutor: PKR

Date	Responsibility	Information	Communication	Critical sense	Self-assessment remarks
			Categories		
16.9.97	B	B	B+	B—	— communicated well — had new info
23.9.97	B	B—	B+	A—	— feel I could have presented more of my own information — could have drawn others in more
30.9.97	B—	N/A*	N/A*	N/A*	— quiet, sort of disjointed — did not really get in tune — brainstorming could be better
7.10.97	D	B—	B	B—	— present in better way — use board — promote deeper understanding — keep asking questions
14.10.97	B+	B	B+	B—	— stayed with topic well — brought up new ideas/ energetic — a good tutorial for me!
21.10.97	B+	A—	B	B+	— lots of information — tried to bring things together — a little more critical sense
28.10.97	A—	B+	B+	B	— should be more critical — need more confidence in presenting info
4.11.97	B+	A—	B+	B+	— good discussion — could use a little more structure — group hesitant to discuss
11.11.97	A—	A—	B+	B	— good tutorial, worked well as a group — felt organized today, good contributions

*N/A = not applicable. This tutorial was unsatisfactory — the tutor had to take charge (see tutor's comments for same day — Figure 4). The student felt that that since the tutor was being so directive, the students had little to do.

Figure 3   Formative evaluation — (Hons.Biology-Pharmacology) student self-assessment

performance over a given period is evaluated by his/her peers. The comments are read out and the tutor, using the criteria given, assigns a grade to each category. The student who is being evaluated has an opportunity to agree or challenge the evaluations done. This procedure is much less traumatic than it seems. If formative

73

Course no.: 3A06		Term: I	Student:		Tutor: PKR
			Categories		
Date	Responsibility	Information	Communication	Critical sense	Self-assessment remarks
16.9.97	B	B	B+	B+	Tried to include everybody, only occasionally got E to contribute
23.9.97	B+	B	B	B+	Better tutorial — did not intervene much — helped discussion of stats — impressed reasons for understanding physiology
30.9.97	A—	B	B	B+	Had to be more directive today — since group not so responsive, lots of gossiping
7.10.97	A—	B	B+	A—	Asked critical questions — helped organizing
14.10.97	A—	B	B	B	Did not participate much — not much need
21.10.97	A	B+	B	B+	Had to be much more active — because discussion on receptors
28.10.97	A—	B	B	B+	Got involved in asking more questions and got them interacting
4.11.97	A—	B	B	A—	Shorter tutorial because of practise TRIPSE. Got them to think though
11.11.97	B+	B	B+	A—	Lots of info covered

Figure 4   Formative evaluation — (Hons.Biology-Pharmacology) tutor self-assessment

evaluation has been carried out appropriately, the summative comments should come as no surprise.

Problem areas

The procedure described above has worked reasonably well. However problems do arise. Though the five specific categories as listed above are not contentious, misunderstanding arises from the descriptors given. There is often little disagreement with the categories labelled information and communication. Students realize very quickly whether or not the information they provide is relevant or useful and whether or not they convey that information clearly. However, the category termed 'critical sense' creates some difficulty. It is important that students learn to evaluate information critically and they can do this not only by referencing their own comments but also by demanding that others provide them as well. The role of the tutor becomes crucial and it is important that they take a more active role by either challenging the students themselves or by persuading them to challenge each other. Clearly, the latter strategy is more useful.

The category termed 'responsibility' is also problematic. In our descriptors, we include active participation as well as listening. Our verbal culture makes it easy for both students and tutors to relate to the active, vocal participant. However the quiet student poses problems. Is the student quiet because she/he is listening actively or silent because they simply have nothing to offer? Several strategies can be adopted. A skilful tutor (or a good group chairperson) can draw out the quiet student and ensure that the others in the group realize the contributions made by a good listener. An alternative is to include a written exercise in the course that could assure the tutor that the quiet student had a grasp of the material. These contributions could then be discussed in the group so that the students realize that the quieter student is functioning well.

ASSESSMENT OF TUTORS BY STUDENTS

It is important that students know that their opinions as the 'consumers' is a mechanism for change. It is also important for the development of tutors that they receive feedback on their performance.

CONCLUSION: THERE IS NO SINGLE RIGHT ANSWER

Problem-based learning is a flexible format where students and tutors are actively engaged in the process of learning. Tutorials are inherently variable and, though there are generic problems, there are no generic solutions. The particular dynamics of the tutorial group, its composition, the level of the students and the experience of the tutors dictate the particular solution to be adopted. In setting up criteria for evaluation, it is important to take the needs of the students and the programme into account. Tutors should make the evaluation process as transparent as possible since the focus is on learning. Tension, suspicion and distrust may be stimulating and challenging under some circumstances but learning is not one of them.

7 HOW TO COPE — A GUIDE FOR STUDENTS

WHAT TO EXPECT — IT IS HARD TO START WITH

Problem-based learning is attractive to students about to emerge from the traditional teacher-centred and didactic experience of schools. Suddenly there is the prospect of learning at your own pace, making your own decisions and accepting responsibility for them.

Impressions at interview

At interview for admission to university the values of the new course are spelled out. The interviewee compares those values with the experience that has been obtained while working at school or college. Of course common sense suggests that there are bound to be snags but, after a short period of adjustment, one expects that all will be well!

It may take 6–12 months to settle in

The reality of problem-based learning courses is somewhat different. The transition from secure, teacher-directed pupil to secure, self-directed adult learner takes longer than one might expect. Six to 12 months is a realistic estimate, although most students have made sufficient progress in the first four to six weeks to recognize the advantages. One must bear in mind that other changes may well be happening at the same time, for example living away from home, having to budget and cope with financial pressures, learning to live with other students, new sexual relationships, and so on.

Causes for discomfort

There are many causes for the initial discomfort. Suddenly being left to decide how and what to learn is like being thrown in to the deep end of a swimming pool without a swimming lesson. Armbands, to prevent drowning, are available — these are the tutors; they are definitely there to help if one is feeling lost.

To the uncertainties of what for many is a completely new approach to learning and the other changes mentioned must be added the new dimension of leaving a school where one's status is secure and joining a much larger group of high achievers in which it is easy to feel anonymous.

Coping with uncertainty

Uncertainty is possibly the greatest problem facing students who are new to problem-based learning. Am I using the right kind of learning resources? Am I learning in sufficient depth? Do I know enough? Do I understand things sufficiently? How am I doing? Some cope better than others with this sort of uncertainty. Being told that being able to cope with uncertainty is an essential ability for all doctors (which is true) is little help!

School learning is guided by a syllabus, supervised by teachers and examined in a series of papers that test factual recall. Students feel that success is the attainment of high grades; simply 'passing' the exam can be reason for disappointment if the next stage in a highly competitive race requires one to be at A grade. It can be stressful but at least one knows what one is supposed to be doing. Now one is faced with what at first appears to be a free-for-all!

There is no 'quick fix' for this problem. Students have to come to terms with a number of realities. It may help to dispel some common myths. One is that the faculty has a clear idea of how much needs to be learned, and is simply not telling the students. Another myth is that if one gets a 'good' tutor, he or she will tell one how much is needed. Students often come to believe there is a hidden curriculum — there is none. The 'reality' of uncertainty is soon discovered in problem-based learning tutorials. One student may say 'I've read this in Guyton'. Another may say 'but in Ganong it says something quite different'. A third textbook is found to differ from both. No one book is right. Merely by discussing these differences and getting used to this type of uncertainty is in fact the main way of accepting and coping with uncertainty.

Uncertainty is commonplace. As a further example, all thinking lay people will accept as obvious (and certain) that infection is the state of being invaded by some foreign organism. However, are we infected if just one micro-organism is present in our system, is the magic number 1,000, or is it some unknown and variable number the size of which depends on the person and the bug? Realizing that there is no right or wrong value is coping with uncertainty!

One positive note is that most students are reassured in the interim by their performance in formative and summative assessments.

SMALL GROUP LEARNING

Need for organization

A tutorial group becomes efficient by identifying what needs to be studied, what resources there are, and by auditing itself. Different groups will be effective in different ways. It is usual in medical problem-based learning courses for the membership of tutorial groups to change every few months (eg at the end of each block of each semester), and as the groups are reformed during the course the previous experience of what worked and what did not is a resource that must be utilized. While this sounds obvious, the skills and discipline needed to achieve it are considerable.

Course book

Instead of a syllabus, one has a course or block book that sets out the general aims of the course, lists the problems to be tackled, identifies some important learning resources, and includes a schedule of timetabled or sign-up events.

Problem order

The course book will contain details of all written problems, along with the order in which they are to be tackled. This order may be important. The course organizers may have specially timetabled demonstrations, displays, lectures or visits to coincide with specific problems, or may have arranged for one or more specialist clinicians to attend the tutorial group in order to answer specialized questions. Changing the order of cases will render useless much organization of resources, and is unwise unless specifically approved by the tutor.

Tackling problems

Having worked through the first four steps of the 7- or 8-step process (chapter 2), the next task is to identify the main learning objectives, which should be determined by (a) the discussion around the problem, and (b) the general aims of the part of the course one is on. A tutor may offer general guidance on the learning objectives or the way that the group is working, but has to be careful not to slip into the old 'chalk and board' information-giving instruction style that problem-based learning is there to replace.

Prioritizing learning objectives

If the problem raises many issues, the group has not only to recognize them but also to rank them in importance. There will certainly not be time to study every single topic in depth.

How much detail is needed?

This topic partly overlaps with the question of uncertainty, discussed above. A recurring question from new students is just how much detail is required if there is no syllabus to refer to. Implicit in the question is the mythical idea that having a syllabus is the answer, even when reflection on school experience reveals that examinations and assessments give only a crude guide, and that students who work hard and obtain more knowledge generally do better than those who attempt the bare minimum. That work ethic applies in problem-based learning. Problem-based learning is not an easy way out; it fosters attitudes and develops communication skills, as well as helping one to acquire knowledge. Problem-based learning should liberate students from the constraints of a syllabus by encouraging them to study topics that interest them in greater depth once the core knowledge has been secured. The course designers have to ensure that the core issues are well covered in the problems, and the students should come to have confidence and the belief in the ability of the group to identify the important issues.

THE TUTORIAL GROUP

Working as part of a group

The individuals in the session must want to act as a group, and to do that they have to show respect for one another even if it seems initially an unpromising exercise. To be functional a group must have, and be seen to value, people with different styles of working. Previous experience and knowledge of individuals can only be used by the group if they are made available; sharing of that kind will only take place in an atmosphere of trust. Trust is also necessary if really meaningful trading of ideas and hypotheses is to occur. The quiet doubt of one participant may allow a receptive group to re-orient its thinking, but a participant is unlikely to offer an idea in the face of ridicule or to colleagues who are persistently too noisy to listen. A tutor can intercede if necessary, but groups become effective by increasingly facilitating their own discussions. Key people are the group leader/chairperson and a secretary/scribe. To be effective, the group leader has to be vigilant that the agenda (the tasks identified in the 7- or 8-step process) is adhered to and that the whole group is participating. The secretary can also focus the flow of ideas if he or she insists that the group thinks deeply enough to condense its thoughts into key phrases or words.

Reviewing the group's strategies

If the tutorial group's initial attempts at problem-based learning are reasonable but clearly could be better, then review the strategy! Students see themselves as radical and free thinking. The reality is that they are more usually ultraconservative, and need a lot of encouragement to change. As a step in the right direction, a group may draw up a 'constitution' based on previous experience to provide firmer guidelines as to how to conduct its business in future. The criteria for success include immediate matters such as completing all the study and reporting objectives they set themselves, and longer-term issues such as the extent to which they missed items that had been identified by other groups or by their tutors. It is essential that the group frequently reviews its progress and actively seeks to improve. The psychological lift that accompanies success helps to drive problem-based learning.

What is the role of the tutor?

The tutor knows in which direction the student is supposed to be going and will give clues to put the student on the right track. The tutor is not there to act as a textbook but can give suggestions, advice and guidance, often by asking questions that make the student re-think things. The tutor may be able to help the student break down big questions into their component parts, and where the student might be able to find information that he or she is seeking.

Remember that the tutor is not witholding information in order to make things difficult for one, but because one has to learn and do things for oneself. After all, no-one can learn or do them on one's behalf.

Need to define and understand terms

Reviewing the *simpler* activities has the most profound effects. We all have a tendency to use terms without defining them and, worse still, we are under the illusion that we know precisely what they mean. Medical students anxious to get to grips with the substantive issues in a problem may not be able to define simple everyday terms such as 'plasma' or 'serum'. They may agree that they all know what the stomach looks like and how big it is, but cannot actually respond there and then to the challenge to produce a sketch with a scale. The omission is all the more bizarre against the ever present question of how much 'detail' is needed. The group has to get to the position of realizing that, unless one can define terms with precision, it is impossible to have a meaningful discussion. Definitions are not details, they are fundamental.

Consensus is not the same as validity

Inexperienced groups may be satisfied that their analysis of a problem has produced agreement. That agreement is somehow the solution. The evidence may make such an agreement appear 'obviously' correct. The need to scrutinize the analysis further may have no appeal. If a group came to the unanimous agreement that the earth was flat, and that the evidence of their own eyes supported that conclusion, they would deserve all the hilarity they provoked in the tutor and course designers. If, however, their consensus was the starting point for examining the hypothesis that the earth was flat, and that they would look for evidence to test it, then they would truly be in the mode of problem-based learning.

Group development

This topic has already been discussed in chapter 5, on tutorial groups, the role of the tutor and the role of individual students. Some additional suggestions come from the University of Newcastle in Australia, which has been at the forefront of development of problem-based learning. Their suggestion is that there are several phases of group development. These are sequential, and groups may get stuck at any phase.

Phase I

One wonders about the rest of the group. Can one trust them? Are they any good? Will one be able to get on with them? How is one going to cope with that nerd for

81

the next six months? Remember that one does not have to love everyone in the group, but one does have to develop a good enough relationship with them to enable one to work together and maintain some sort of flow of activities. One is not living with them, just trying to learn with them!

Phase 2

A degree of vigorous competition emerges between the various group members, sometimes at the level of intense debate and at other times degenerating into bickering. This generally settles down as members of the group come to appreciate the strengths and contributions of each other, and as the group settles down to the task that confronts them rather than competing with each other. Occasionally groups get locked in to this argumentative phase, and much of the discussion consists of debasing and devaluing the contributions of others. If this does happen, it is a good idea to discuss the problem openly with the group and seek help from the tutor or other members of staff.

Phase 3

Once these stages are left behind, the group settles down and gets on with its work. From time to time, old problems may re-emerge. These are generally recognizable from their symptoms: absenteeism, lateness, failure to carry out agreed work, non-productive arguing, splitting of the group, quiet sessions, and discontent. If this happens to one's group, remember to stop and devote some time to the health and development of the group itself. Groups enhance the processes and value of learning from working through problems, but if that is not what is happening in one's group, something is wrong and one needs to take time out to resolve the problem.

PERSONAL LEARNING AND STUDYING STRATEGIES

How and from whom should one learn?

In a problem-based learning course there are few sessions in which a teacher tells one what he or she wants and one has no role other than to listen. In a problem-based learning course *the student* decides what needs to be learnt about, and why, rather than a teacher telling one what he or she thinks one wants to know. One has to adopt an active role and take responsibility for ones own learning. One determines what one wants to know, why one needs to know it, and one appraises each piece of information critically and stores it within an appropriate place in one's memory. One has to learn to use 'teachers' as resources, being prepared to question them, interact with them, and evaluate their information (it may be incorrect!).

How should one change?

Faced with a major change in the way one learns, one should not be afraid to change ones personal study habits. One should rethink ones approach rather than trying to redesign the course! As with the group process, one should review what one is doing and see if it fits with the problem-based learning activities that one is pursuing. If the old routines delivered the examination grades at school, it is undeniably tempting to persist with them, even in the face of ones own experience that they no longer deliver.

Whereas in a conventional course one can sometimes survive despite leaving all one's study to the last few days before an examination, this strategy is guaranteed to fail in a problem-based learning course.

How much time should one spend on study?

It is helpful to keep a diary of how much time one spends on personal study and, particularly, how that time is distributed between the various themes and issues the group have elected to cover. The truth usually hurts: most of us either put less time in than we believe or concentrate on easier topics at the expense of more challenging ones.

How hard should one be working?

This is difficult to answer, partly because individual students have differing 'learning efficiency'. Some are better than others at focusing in on topics, and some are better at being sure of their facts than others. When one goes to the supermarket, is it best to have a shopping list, or can one manage just by ambling past the shelves hoping for inspiration and picking items that one fancies? Some students are highly organized, head for the library with a clear 'shopping list' of issues to be sorted out, and can cover a lot of ground. Others are less well focused, and end up reading large volumes of material without being quite sure of the purpose.

83

The plain fact is that if one goes out every evening and weekend, then however great one's learning efficiency, insufficient time is being spent on studying. It has been estimated that students require a minimum of 16 hours independent study per week for a problem-based learning medical course. In theory this can be achieved in the working day, but in practise this is near impossible. Although the medical course in the UK lasts six years (including a one year pre-medical course for biology, physics and chemistry), in north America there are medical courses that last only three years. There are two main differences. One is that the medical students in north America are graduates, having already obtained a degree (not necessarily in a subject connected with medicine). The other is that the north American students spend far more time (in some cases in the order of 100 hours a week) studying; in some medical schools, if one is looking for a student one rings the library not the student's home!

Problem-based learning is no shortcut. Students on old (ie conventional) courses had to work some evenings and weekends, and problem-based learning does not diminish the need to work.

Exploring topics of personal interest

Although a group has agreed to specific learning objectives, there is still scope for an individual to pursue an additional topic of special interest. Ones own curiosity and urge to follow something through may also benefit the rest of the group.

It is healthy to focus on difficulties

Students engaged in problem-based learning may seem to be unduly concerned with the difficulties they are having in understanding the topics. It is healthy and normal to be questioning what one is doing. On more conventional courses, progress appears to be smoother as such questioning (if it occurs at all) is postponed to the pre-examination revision period.

The real world is not cut and dried

One can be assured that success is near with problem-based learning when one accepts as a matter of fact that the textbooks are often, like progress reports, only partially accurate, and when one no longer hears oneself ask what is *the* answer to a question.

IS PROBLEM-BASED LEARNING SUITABLE FOR EVERYONE?

It should be

This is a bit like asking if all 18-year-olds are adults (in the sense of being self-directed). The answer is that some are more ready than others, and any medical school that uses problem-based learning must be prepared to help students through the transition from a state of dependency to a more independent existence. The fact is that school education (at least in the UK) is changing, and self-direction has become much more a feature of school programmes than used to be the case.

Personality types who may have special problems

In theory, problem-based learning should be suitable for anyone and everyone. In practise, however, we recognize two groups who may experience special difficulty in the transition process. One is the very dependent teenager, who relies almost totally on teachers and parents for direction and instruction, and who becomes lost without constant guidance. The other is the very bright school child who has achieved the very highest grades and who has sailed effortlessly through every examination without ever having faced the slightest challenge or difficulty. We have come across a small number of such individuals who have been unable to cope with the relative lack of direction and uncertainty of a problem-based learning course. Indeed there are a handful of problem-based learning medical schools who try, through their selection process, to take only students who have already shown the capacity to overcome some sort of important challenge or hurdle in life.

8 HOW TO COPE—A GUIDE FOR STAFF

Most people entering problem-based learning as tutors have previously learned and taught solely on conventional courses. This chapter is intended to help staff facing this change. The tutor's role is also discussed in chapter 5, and inevitably there is some overlap between that exposition of the various tutor roles and the advice given here. What is written here is no substitute for proper courses designed to train tutors, and no-one should try to tutor on a problem-based learning course without having attended an appropriate staff development training programme.

CHANGING TO PROBLEM-BASED LEARNING — A MAJOR UPHEAVAL

Changing to problem-based learning is a big change for students, but an even greater adjustment for tutors who come from a conventional educational system. Yet in many respects the problem-based learning approach formalizes ideas that good teachers have used for years. We all aspire to introduce students to the fascination we have for our subject, and the satisfaction we get from answering questions that at first seemed too complicated to resolve. Our motivation is derived from curiosity and the freedom to explore. We have developed an instinct as adult learners to break problems down into manageable tasks and to question the sense of the solutions as they emerge. As a result we have acquired a corpus of knowledge that the next generation of students is expected to acquire. The rules of that game are familiar, except that now someone has apparently rewritten the rule book.

What problem-based learning liberates us to do is to teach the skills of learning rather than plough through the corpus of facts.

EXPECTATIONS FROM EXPERIENCE OF CONVENTIONAL EDUCATION

What is a tutor? How is one supposed to conduct a tutorial or lecture? Answers to those questions may produce a variety of emphases, but they would probably all have in common the notion of the tutor being an expert able to impart knowledge.

Ideally, perhaps, the tutor could be a role model, enthusiastically communicating a considered analysis of the subject. On a more pragmatic level there is the element of control, control that inevitably extended to setting an agenda that one could cope with. Much of that description of conventional teaching activity sounds perfectly reasonable. Being an enthusiast of long standing helps a teacher to distil into a lecture, information that may be difficult to access through library books.

In a tutorial, a more open-ended forum, one will have felt secure to a degree. Matters of knowledge and interpretation are likely to have fallen within ones sphere. Whether or not one was lecturing or tutoring there was always a syllabus as a guide, maybe even knowledge that specific topics are on an examination paper and must be covered. The students were there to be taught and in a number of ways the teacher was their resource. Everyone knew where they were and where they were likely to be at specified times of the teaching year. Even the realization that one would probably be disappointed once again with the limited recall and understanding of the gems of information one laid before the students was bearable: one knew that one had done one's bit, and the appropriate facts had been presented.

Problem-based learning offers an apparently high risk strategy as an alternative learning scheme. The students are to be given the responsibility for their learning, so where does that leave the tutor, his/her expertise and his/her enthusiasm? How can anyone ensure that the students learn all they need to know?

THE REALITY

The old course

One of the more surprising revelations about change is the degree to which it endows the old course with qualities that in truth it never had. There are undoubtedly merits in the traditional chalk-and-board teaching. These did not include the accurate transfer of information from the notes of the lecturer to the mind of the student. Neither could the old courses be relied on to foster curiosity, surely one attribute we would all like our students to develop. Passing on large amounts of information by didactic teaching, and then expecting students promptly to analyse it and really learn the key facts and arguments was never realistic. The temptation was to store all of the newly acquired information,

87

including errors of transcription and omissions, and to revise it at a later date, most frequently just before examinations. With that pressure, students were always tempted to second guess the examiners and spot likely topics and disregard the rest. It was also more difficult to cut across the compartments that each batch of lecture notes became in order to integrate topics that were related in content but separated in time. It was commonplace for students to find that their prime source of revision material was notes made at lectures that had never been subsequently corrected or reinforced by textbook reading.

If the learning methods were faulty, this was overshadowed by an even greater problem, the discipline-specific examination steeplechase, studying from one hurdle to the next, memorizing and forgetting a huge amount of information at each step. When it came to the job for which one had been trained, almost all of this basic information had been lost.

If information transfer by lecture is so inefficient why persist with it? If students get an appreciation of the facts and their interrelations in small group tutorials, and get turned on by literature and research projects, it is sensible to make greater use of those strategies.

The problem-based learning course

The appeal of this style of learning is that it offers choice and the responsibility to the student who is free within a given frame of reference to be curious. Tutors have been involved in designing the problems and stand back to keep a watchful eye on progress. Problem-based learning gives students that opportunity throughout the course but, in order for the student to be successful, tutors have to design cases or problems that do provide frames of reference and then stand back to be supportive. Both designing workable cases and allowing students to use them in their own way are demanding tasks, especially the latter.

THE TUTOR AS A FACILITATOR OF LEARNING

Need for encouragement and guidance

If students are to tackle problems that have been carefully constructed to meet overall learning objectives, they will need encouragement, guidance and support, particularly in the early stages. The role of the tutor is crucial. Students testify to the importance of getting a flying, confidence-inspiring start. A confidence deflating tutor might be tolerated by experienced practitioners, but is poison to students who are new to problem-based learning.

Need for real support for the course

As with any form of teaching, the tutor has to believe in the process. Students can cope with error and differences in style but they should not be expected to deal with negativity from tutors. 'If the faculty don't believe in what they are doing, why should we?'. For new tutors who are in reality keen on the course, uncertainties about their new responsibilities can be misinterpreted.

Need to resist the urge to teach

The desire to slip into the old habits of didactic teaching under the guise of helping the group is often overwhelming, and it must be resisted at all costs! Novice tutors have been known to leave their lecture notes from the old course with their students, and have been seen delivering mini (and sometimes not so mini) lectures. There are times when, if the group gets stuck, the tutor can usefully intervene during group discussions, but it should be to ask a constructive question, supply advice or an occasional nugget of information, in order to get the discussion restarted. Observing discussions in progress shows that frequent intervention by a tutor is very disruptive. The tutor who says just enough to show that he/she is on the students' side may be seen as very supportive — 'he'd say something if we were going off at a tangent'.

Need to allow students to make mistakes and learn from them

Students have to be allowed to make mistakes, and to learn from them. A frustration for tutors is the feeling that their group is missing the point or failing to make the connections that the course design team had in mind. What may appear obvious to the experienced eye (ie the tutor) is clearly not always obvious to the uninitiated, but students have to learn by trial and error. Keeping quiet (and avoiding signalling by body language) long enough for that to happen is a discipline that tutors have to develop. What is exhilarating to the tutors is the realization that their group are actually mastering the method.

89

Need to support to help maintain momentum

Supportive comments on general progress, and reminders if there has been no attention given at all to certain aspects of the case, serve to maintain momentum and, with that, confidence and enthusiasm.

HELPING A DYSFUNCTIONAL GROUP

Watching a good group in action is breathtaking, but what does one do with a group that appears to be dysfunctional? It is of prime importance that the group should believe that it is not intrinsically bad and unable to work together effectively. The problem to solve here, as in real life, is sorting out what is going wrong. The skills exercised in the process are one of the benefits of the problem-based learning method. The group may feel it is being dominated by particular individuals, or is "carrying" individuals who do not contribute to its work. A vigilant tutor should encourage the group to analyse its activities and recognize that their first impressions are not always accurate, and certainly bear as much examination as the academic content of the problem. Individual students may feel that they are having an unwanted role thrust on them, and are relieved to talk it through with someone.

Avoid blaming the group or the course

Difficulties may arise with the strategies that students have adopted for group or individual study. If they are not as successful as expected, the blame may be placed with the 'group'. If the difficulties are not resolved, the perception may grow that their roots lie in the problem-based learning course and would not have been encountered on a traditional course! That refuge is also tempting for tutors who feel they are not coping.

Anxiety can be healthy

Perverse as it may appear, student and tutor anxiety arise from one of the strengths of problem-based learning, namely that it requires the participants to constantly question how effective they are at what they are doing. Traditional courses will have no difficulties en route because, in general, difficulties are not sought. Staff and students both have their post mortems at the 'appropriate' place, the end of the course.

The tutor as a subject expert

If a problem happens to be narrowly focused on a single discipline (eg pharmacology of a drug in someone who has taken an overdose) then the tutor can act as both facilitator of student discussions and, if needed, as an expert resource. For multidisciplinary courses like preclinical medicine, tutors are less likely to wear both hats. Tutors can hardly be experts in all components of the course. However in the design of cases, and for students who want advice on specific matters within a tutor's area of expertise, the tutor's subject specific expertise is required. In the design and marking of assessments, problem-based learning like any other type of higher education course needs experts. If a problem is likely to need the help of an expert, this need should be anticipated at the planning stage, and arrangements made for this expertise to be available to students if their own tutor is not an appropriate expert. One way to manage this resource is to timetable the expert to attend the feedback tutorial, to deal with specific queries that are produced by the students. Such experts need to be in tune with the ethos of problem-based learning and have an understanding of the process. Being a subject expert may be a diasadvantage if it leads to the tutor saying too much too soon.

TUTOR'S ROLE IN COURSE DESIGN

Tutors should have the opportunity to join a problem-based learning planning and management group, to gain an insight into the challenges of course and problem design. The design of problem material is hard but stimulating work. It can be a sobering experience to find that ones hobby horses of the old course are discarded in the design of the new one. If a case integrates topics that were formerly presented by colleagues from different disciplines, the staff are exposed first hand to the kind of group activity that the students will experience. Staff development is a valuable consequence of the whole process. The multidisciplinary nature of this planning and management process means that one comes to work with colleagues from a different discipline who in a conventional course would have only been known by name.

9 HOW TO DESTROY PROBLEM-BASED LEARNING — AVOIDABLE SERIOUS PITFALLS

This chapter contains details of lethal pitfalls, all of which the authors have seen in practice and must be avoided at all cost.

NOT UNDERSTANDING HOW PROBLEM-BASED LEARNING WORKS

If students are to get the best out of problem-based learning, they have to understand how and why it works. The steps of the tutorial process operate best if one understands why the steps are there. It follows that students should not be launched straight in to a problem-based learning course without some explanation of how it works. It is common to find that a dysfunctional or disaffected student has no idea of how problem-based learning works or why it is used, and consequently feels that the method is being 'imposed'. Helping students and staff to understand problem-based learning was the major impetus for this book.

PROBLEMS RESULTING FROM POOR PLANNING

Insufficient study time

In a problem-based learning course, there must be sufficient free time in the timetable to allow students the opportunity for independent study. There is no point of students attending regular problem-based learning tutorial sessions if they have a fully-packed timetable for the rest of the week. Those who plan problem-based learning courses must allow students adequate time to tackle their learning objectives.

Inappropriate examinations

The wrong type of assessments can wreck a whole course. The very best problem-based learning course will fail if it is undermined by an examination system which simply tests the ability of students to cram large amounts of useless knowledge into short-term memory.

92

PROBLEMS ARISING IN TUTORIALS

Re-arranging the order of problems

If the order of problems has been carefully designed by the planners, for example so that specific experts can be made available to coincide with the discussion of individual topics, then re-arranging the order in which cases are discussed is disruptive. The tutor should be able to advise on the wisdom or otherwise of changing the order of problems.

Bypassing steps 2–4 of the tutorial process

Some students (usually as a result of encouragement by a poorly trained tutor) simply read through the problem, and then spend a few minutes deciding on what topics to study. For example, in one case the group, having read through the problem, decided they were unfamiliar with the topics of routine antenatal care, screening in pregnancy and morning sickness, and they agreed the best thing they could do was read up on these topics.

Failing to engage in the steps of the tutorial process (as listed in chapter 2) means that one is failing to access (a) one's own, and (b) the group's prior knowledge. Failing to 'have a go' at brainstorming makes subsequent reading much less productive, and much less information is likely to be retained.

Being insufficiently critical

Much information in textbooks is incorrect. The same applies to information provided by staff or fellow students. An essential task is to evaluate the reliability of information. When a member of the group offers an item of information, a reflex action should be to ask 'how do I know this is true?'. Frequent questions during tutorial groups should be questions to evaluate information, such as 'what is the evidence for that statement?', or more simply 'what is the source of that information?'. One should get in the habit of giving the source of one's information. There is a big difference between 'I think I once read somewhere that...' and 'a paper in last week's *Lancet* demonstrated that...'. Never uncritically accept information, even if it comes from a senior member of staff. Do not be frightened of asking staff this sort of question; one of the most enjoyable aspects of teaching is having one's assumptions and statements challenged. It is often the searching question from a student that can make one completely re-think a topic,

93

which can be very refreshing. Unreliable 'experts' instantly give themselves away, by irritation or obvious bluffing. A greater degree of tact is needed when pressing a fellow student for his or her source of information, as it can be rather threatening to be challenged in this way.

Consensus is not in itself a satisfactory end-product

A group of students come together in a new problem-based learning group, and a few weeks later as a result of discussion, they achieve consensus. Students commonly equate consensus with critical appraisal, which are as far apart as the north and south poles. Critical appraisal is not a form of agreement but a type of questioning — what is the evidence, how reliable is the evidence, is the evidence consistent with other information, and do sources of information agree? It is more useful to identify and understand areas of disagreement than to achieve consensus. Consensus can be dangerously seductive. Take the following true example, where the problem centred around alcoholic cirrhosis, gastric acid and bleeding oesophageal varices. The students concluded:

'It is normal to have veins in the oesophagus. They get eroded by drinking alcohol. Because they get eroded the vein wall weakens, the vein bleeds, and blood pours out'.

That consensus should have become a hypothesis, to be followed by evidence (and not just argument) that supports or refutes the hypothesis.

Producing excessively broad learning objectives

This is usually the result of inadequate brainstorming or a superficial discussion. In the case of John Smythe, who had a rapidly fatal illness (see chapter 2), a poorly functioning group might decide simply to read all about meningococcal infection. A better group would have some clearly focused themes, such as why do meningococcal infections cause purpura, why and how do they produce a rapidly fatal illness, what is the significance of fever in this illness, and was this child's death preventable and, if so, how?

Splitting main learning tasks

Some groups (usually as a result of poor tutoring) divide all their learning tasks. Each member of the group is given a different major learning objective to study and, at the second tutorial, each student gives a short presentation of what he or she has found. What happens is: (i) most students fail to address the majority of the core learning objectives; (ii) the group then dozes while individual students attempt to give mini-lectures on their own individual topics; and (iii) the whole group loses the value of synthesizing different perspectives into a common understanding. An essential feature of problem-based learning is that the group agrees an achievable list of core learning objectives that are all tackled by every member of the group.

There is, however, no objection to individuals identifying and pursuing peripheral learning objectives. This can be done formally as part of the group process, so that each student identifies, and reports back, on say one peripheral issue in addition to the core issues. The objective need not necessarily be a major or time-consuming one; it might just involve looking something up in a couple of books or asking a doctor. Local experience has been that giving individuals their own unique assignments may help to motivate certain individuals, who feel responsible and respected by the group when entrusted with an assignment. Individual assignments may also encourage some quiet or shy members of a group to contribute.

Poorly trained or untrained tutors

Students and tutorials stand little chance of good function if tutors are untrained or dysfunctional. Examples of seriously dysfunctional tutoring are failure to attend, dominance, negativism, giving mini-lectures, or telling the students to bypass the steps of the tutorial process. Students have a responsibility to report to the faculty those tutors who fail to attend, who are disruptive, or who are seriously dysfunctional in any way.

NOT DOING ENOUGH WORK

Being a brilliant tutorial group member is not enough

Problem-based learning has many virtues, but being a substitute for work is not one of them! Problem-based learning is not a short-cut to knowledge. However well the tutorial group is functioning, the benefits will not be reaped without individual study relating to the agreed learning objectives. In our experience, the single most common error is quite simply failure to work hard enough, and probably the most common cause of this is a failure to realize just how much effort is required to make a real success of the undergraduate course.

10 DOES PROBLEM-BASED LEARNING WORK AND, IF SO, HOW?

A detailed discussion of this topic is beyond the scope of this book, and this chapter is only a brief outline. In short, the justification for problem-based learning lies in its compatibility with the principles of adult education and cognitive psychology [27], evidence of efficacy in certain areas, and absence of the major drawbacks of traditional medical curricula [28] (Table 1).

TABLE I SOME DRAWBACKS OF TRADITIONAL CURRICULA
• create an artificial divide between basic science and clinical medicine
• time is wasted acquiring knowledge that is subsequently forgotten or found to be irrelevant
• application of the acquired knowledge can be difficult
• acquisition and retention of information that has no apparent relevance can be boring and demoralising for students
• strong focus on individual disciplines

ADVANTAGES OF PROBLEM-BASED LEARNING

Most students enjoy the active participation which problem-based learning fosters, and consider the process to be relevant, stimulating and fun [29,30]. The learning environment created by problem-based learning is more convivial for students and teachers as traditional barriers between students and faculty are reduced [31]. Problem-based learning fosters self-directed learning skills [9,32–35] which, in turn, is likely to lead to medical graduates becoming life-long learners [35–37]. Problem-based learning promotes deeper rather than superficial learning [38–40]. Problem-based learning activities bring together staff from different disciplines, initially in planning and developing the course and later in tutoring and assessments, promoting interaction between basic scientists and clinicians. Finally, problem-based learning enhances motivation and helps the development of interpersonal skills.

HOW DOES PROBLEM-BASED LEARNING WORK?

There is evidence that problem-based learning achieves five main objectives [27]. These are listed overleaf.

Structuring of knowledge

Several studies demonstrate that students in undergraduate problem-based learning curricula integrate their knowledge of basic science concepts into clinical problems better than students in conventional curricula [39,41–43]. An emphasis on patient problems is believed to have this effect by integrating basic and clinical sciences. Clinical performance and skills of students exposed to problem-based learning are superior to those of students from traditional curricula [29]. A possible explanation is that learning arises from patient problems; this helps to integrate clinical and basic science knowledge. A critical issue is not 'greater knowledge' but the *quality* of knowledge. Through problem-based learning, students are likely to acquire knowledge that is relevant to clinical problems, gain a deeper understanding and so better remember and recall the information.

Development of an effective clinical reasoning process

Hmelo *et al* compared the effects of a problem-based learning course and a traditional course on problem solving [44,45]. The results showed greater use of hypothesis-driven reasoning in the problem-based learning group and a greater coherence in the learners' explanations.

There is often confusion between problem-based learning and learning about *problem solving*. It is important to differentiate between the two. Problem solving skills appear to be content- or knowledge-specific. The more you know, the better you are at solving problems. There is no evidence for a problem solving skill that is independent of knowledge. Thus, problem-based learning helps the development of clinical reasoning solely by improving knowledge. There is no evidence that problem-based learning curricula (or any other curricula for that matter) are able to enhance students' problem solving skills independent of their acquisition of knowledge [32].

Improving retention of information

Reviewing the published work for evidence supporting the theoretical advantages of problem-based learning, Norman and Schmidt [32] noted the observation in several studies that problem-based learning learners retain knowledge much better than students receiving conventional teaching. Problem-based learning leads to better recall of information for three reasons [13]. First, mobilization of previous

97

knowledge simulates learners to construct explanatory models, and this facilitates the processing and comprehension of new information. Second, new information is better understood if learners are stimulated to elaborate on it. Elaboration in problem-based learning can take several forms, such as discussion, note-taking or answering questions. Third, learning in context makes information more accessible for later use.

Development of self-directed learning skills

Self-directed learning skills refer to being able to identify own learning needs and locate appropriate resources. Work by Blumberg and Michael supports the hypothesis that problem-based learning enhances self-directed learning skills [33]. During both preclinical and clinical clerkship years, problem-based learning students borrowed more material from the library than students from a conventional curriculum. In another study, graduates from a problem-based learning curriculum, after being in a position to observe the performance of graduates from conventional curricula, viewed themselves as better prepared in independent learning skills, problem solving and self evaluation techniques as compared to graduates from conventional curricula [29]. Both studies demon-strated that problem-based learning does have a large and potentially long lasting impact on self directed learning skills.

Increasing motivation for learning

The student-centred learning approach of problem-based learning increases motivation because students themselves define the learning issues and decide for themselves what is relevant for their learning [9]. In addition, discussion of problems enhances intrinsic interest in subject matter because it involves the learners more actively in the issues at hand [46].

REFERENCES

1. Clandfield D, Sivell J, eds. *Cooperative Learning and Social Change. Selected Writings of Célestin Freinet.* Toronto: Our Schools/Our Selves Education Foundation, 1990.

2. Harris JW, Horrigan DL, Ginther JR, Ham TH. Pilot study in teaching hematology with emphasis on self-education by the students. *J Med Educat* 1962; **37**: 719–36.

3. Ham TH. Medical education at Western Reserve University. A progress report for the sixteen years, 1946–1962. *N Engl J Med* 1962; **267**: 868–74.

4. Echt R, Chan SW. A new problem–oriented and student–centred curriculum at Michigan State University. *J Med Educat* 1977; **52**: 681–3.

5. Neufeld VR, Barrows HS. The 'McMaster philosophy': an approach to medical education. *J Med Educat* 1974; **49**: 1040–50.

6. Walsh W. The development of the McMaster programme in medical education. *Br J Hosp Med* 1973; **12**: 722–30.

7. Hamilton JD. The McMaster curriculum: a critique. *BMJ* 1976; **1**: 1191–6.

8. Barrows HS, Abrahamson S. The programmed patient: a technique for appraising student performance in clinical neurology. *J Med Educat* 1964; **39**: 802–5.

9. Barrows HS, Tamblyn RM. *Problem–Based Learning. An Approach to Medical Education.* New York: Springer Publishing Company, 1980.

10. David TJ, Patel L. Adult learning theory, problem based learning, and paediatrics. *Arch Dis Child* 1995; **73**: 357–63.

11. Regehr G, Norman GR. Issues in cognitive psychology: implications for professional education. *Acad Med* 1996; **71**: 988–1001.

12. Tulving E, Thomson DM. Encoding specificity and retrieval processes in episodic memory. *Psychol Rev* 1973; **80**: 352–73.

13. Schmidt HG. Foundations of problem–based learning: some explanatory notes. *Med Educ* 1993; **27**: 422–32.

14. Gijselaers WH, Schmidt HG. Development and evaluation of a causal model of problem–based learning. In: Nooman ZM, Schmidt HG, Ezzat ES, eds. *Innovation in medical education: an evaluation of its present status.* New York: Springer Publishing Company, 1990: 95–113.

15. Glick TH, Armstrong EG. Crafting cases for problem–based learning: experience in a neuroscience course. *Med Educ* 1996; **30**: 24–30.

16. Dolmans DHJM, Gijselaers WH, Schmidt HG, Van der Meer SB. Problem effectiveness in a course using problem–based learning. *Acad Med* 1993; **68**: 207–13.

17. Dolmans D. How Students Learn in a Problem-based Curriculum. Limburg: University of Limburg, 1994. PhD thesis

18. Brown G, Atkins M. *Anonymous, Effective Teaching in Higher Education.* London: Routledge, 1988: 50–90

19. Barrows H S. *The Tutorial Process.* Springfield, Illinois: Southern Illinois University School of Medicine, 1992.

20. Hitchcock MA, Anderson AS. Dealing with dysfunctional tutorial groups. *Teach Learn Med* 1997; **9**: 19–24.

21. Blake JM, Norman GR, Smith EK. Report card from McMaster: student evaluation at a problem–based medical school. *Lancet* 1995; **345**: 899–902.

22. Patel L, David TJ. Everybody has won, and all must have prizes. *Lancet* 1996; **348**: 1497.

23. David TJ, Patel L. Adult learning theory, prizes and motivation: fundamental learning issues. In: Scherpbier AJJA, Van der Vleuten CPM, Rethans JJ, Van der Steeg AFW, eds. *Advances in Medical Education*. Dordrecht: Kluwer Academic Publishers, 1997: 7–10.

24. Gerstenberger HJ, Davis JH. Report of a case of anaphylaxis following an intradermal protein sensitization test. *JAMA* 1921; **76**: 721–3.

25. Case SM. Assessment truths that we hold as self–evident and their implications. In: Scherpbier AJJA, Van der Vleuten CPM, Rethans JJ, Van der Steeg AFW, eds. *Advances in Medical Education*. Dordrecht: Kluwer Academic Publishers, 1997: 2–6.

26. Blake JM, Norman GR, Keane DR *et al*. Introducing progress testing in McMaster University's problem–based medical curriculum: psychometric properties and effect on learning. *Acad Med* 1996; **71**: 1002–7.

27. Dolmans D, Schmidt H. The advantages of problem–based curricula. *Postgrad Med J* 1996; **72**: 535–8.

28. Finuncane PM, Johnson SM, Prideaux DJ. Problem–based learning: its rationale and efficacy. *Med J Aust* 1998; **168**: 445–8.

29. Albanese MA, Mitchell S. Problem–based learning: a review of literature on its outcomes and implementation issues. *Acad Med* 1993; **68**: 52–81.

30. Des Marchais JE. A student–centred, problem–based curriculum: 5 years' experience. *Can Med Assoc J* 1993; **148**: 1567–72.

31. Blight J. Problem based, small group learning: an idea whose time has come. *BMJ* 1995; **311**: 342–3.

32. Norman GR, Schmidt HG. The psychological basis of problem–based learning: a review of the evidence. *Acad Med* 1992; **67**: 557–65.

33. Blumberg P, Michael JA. Development of self–directed learning behaviours in a partially teacher–directed problem–based learning curriculum. *Teach Learn Med* 1992; **4**: 3–8.

34. Dolmans DHJM, Schmidt HG. What drives the student in problem–based learning? *Med Educ* 1994; **28**: 280–372.

35. Shin JH, Haynes RB, Johnson ME. The effect of problem–based, self–directed undergraduate education on lifelong learning. *Can Med Assoc J* 1993; **148**: 969–76.

36. Donner RS, Bickley H. Problem–based learning in American medical education: an overview. *Bull Med Libr Assoc* 1993; **81**: 294–8.

37. Headrick L, Kaufman A, Stillman P *et al*. Teaching and learning methods for new generalist physicians. *J Gen Intern Med* 1994; **9**(suppl 1): S42–9.

38. Engel CE. Problem–based learning. *Br J Hosp Med* 1992; **48**: 325–9.

39. Vernon DTA, Blake RL. Does problem–based learning work? A meta–analysis of evaluative research. *Acad Med* 1993; **68**: 550–63.

40. Newble DI, Clarke RM. The approaches to learning of students in a traditional and in an innovative problem–based medical school. *Med Educ* 1986; **20**: 267–73.

41. Patel VL, Groen GJ, Norman GR. Effects of conventional and problem–based medical curricula on problem solving. *Acad Med* 1991; **66**: 380–9.
42. Hmelo CE. *Development of independent learning and thinking: a study of medical problem solving and problem–based learning.* Nashville, Tennessee: Vanderbilt University, 1994. Unpublished doctoral dissertation.
43. Schmidt H, Machiels–Bongaerts M, Hermans H *et al.* The development of diagnostic competence: comparison of a problem–based, an integrated, and a conventional medical curriculum. *Acad Med* 1996; **71**: 658–64.
44. Hmelo CE, Gotterer GS, Bransford JD. A theory–driven approach to assessing the cognitive effects of problem based learning. *Instr Sci* 1997; **25**: 387–408.
45. Hmelo CE. Cognitive consequences of problem–based learning for the early development of medical expertise. *Teach Learn Med* 1998; **10**: 92–100.
46. Schmidt HG. Intrinsic motivation and achievement: two exploratory studies. *Pedagogische Studien* 1983; **60**: 385–95.

INDEX